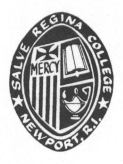

THE · GIFT · OF

_____

THE
LAST
CRUSADE

THE
LAST
CRUSADE

The War on Consumption

1862–1954

MARK CALDWELL

ATHENEUM

New York

1988

Copyright © 1988 by Mark Caldwell

Atheneum
Macmillan Publishing Company
866 Third Avenue, New York, N.Y. 10022
Collier Macmillan Canada, Inc.

Library of Congress Cataloging-in-Publication Data
Caldwell, Mark.
    The last crusade: the war on consumption, 1862-1954 / by Mark Caldwell.
    p. cm.
    Bibliography: p.
    Includes index.
    ISBN 0-689-11810-4
    1. Tuberculosis—History. I. Title.
RC310.C35 1988
614.5'42'09—dc 19   87-23090
                                                                    CIP

Macmillan books are available at special discounts
for bulk purchases
for sales promotions, premiums, fund-raising, or educational use.
For details, contact:

Special Sales Director
Macmillan Publishing Company
866 Third Avenue
New York, N.Y. 10022

10 9 8 7 6 5 4 3 2 1

Printed in the United States of America

He was dropsical, he was consumptive, he was surfeited, was gouty, and, as some say, he had a tang of the Pox in his bowels. Yet the Captain of all these men of death that came against him to take him away was the Consumption, for 'twas that that brought him down to the grave.

—John Bunyan
The Life and Death of Mr. Badman

The patients who did well at the sanatorium, and that was the vast majority, remember it with great fondness. Why? Well, I think most of them went home realizing things that they thought were terribly important were not, and things they thought were not important were.

—Dr. Gordon Meade
last director of the Trudeau Sanatorium
Saranac Lake, New York

Acknowledgments

I would like to thank James L. Kurtz, whose hospitality in the Adirondacks first introduced me to the landscape from which America's War on Consumption was launched; Dr. Gordon Meade, for his generosity both with time and information; David Kirstein, for guiding me through Saranac Lake and its history; and Steve Saletan, M.D., who combed my manuscript for medical howlers (he found many; I take responsibility for any remaining).

Thanks are also due to Louise Bishop, Robert Cornfield, Janet P. Decker, James Earl, David Ekstrom, Anne MacDonald Evans, Steve Evans, Gary Giddins, Constance Hassett, Helen Jarvis, Drew Jewett, Walter Kendrick, Dinah Knot, Susan Leon, Jim Mann, Barbara Parnass, Ann Rittenberg, Charles Schlessiger, Christian R. Sporck, Ruth Stern, Frances Toone, Dr. Francis Trudeau, and Marshall Watson.

Nor could the book have been written without the cooperation of the New York Academy of Medicine and its staff, the Trudeau Institute, the Saranac Lake Free Library, the Metropolitan Life Insurance Company, the American Lung Association, and Historic Saranac Lake.

Finally, I owe a debt of gratitude to Fordham University for its generous support.

Contents

THE
LAST
CRUSADE

Introduction

This is a work of medical history by a literary critic. As such it is less a study of dramatic discoveries and evolving scientific theories than a retelling of stories, some long forgotten, and a history of images, many never before explored. I am interested in what people—all kinds of people—thought about tuberculosis, how they pictured it and wrote about it, from the time the American public first discovered consumption as a national scourge, in the 1870s, until it finally went down to partial defeat under the onslaught of new antibiotics in the 1950s.

Scientists, of course, loom large in the history of this crusade. Toward the close of the 1800s, as they stood on the brink of a century of major achievements, it was perhaps their fiercest challenge, the Great Killer, the White Plague. If they could unravel its mysteries and repair its ravages, science, still in many ways a marginal pursuit, might advance from its status as a gentlemanly but slightly eccentric pastime to become a major social force. And, naturally, doctors (by no means all of whom were scientists) played a central role. As healers their authority stood at risk—how could they claim respect for their art if they remained ignorant and impotent before the world's leading cause of death, the disease that was, by some estimates, carrying off a third of the human race?

But tuberculosis was more than a scientist's obsession or a challenge to physicians. In the United States it became a national preoccupation and the pivot for a miniature economy. Businessmen, small and grand, built empires on it. Towns, like Saranac Lake, New York, grew up around the treatment of tuberculosis, throve during the heyday of the sanatorium cure, and withered afterward. Health crusaders inundated the nation with a flood of antituberculosis propaganda—exhibits, pamphlets, novels, films, broadcasts, Christmas seals, billboards, mass mailings, publicity blitzes. Novelists and playwrights turned the disease into imaginative literature; charlatans turned it into fast cash; crackpots turned it into macabre comedy. Social reformers, devising strategies to combat tuberculosis, formulated policies that helped shape the cities we live in today: codes governing air, space, and light, enacted at the close of the nineteenth century, were much influenced by contemporary notions about what impeded the spread of consumption.

Scientists and mountebanks, opportunists and philanthropists, visionaries and lunatics—all drew attention to themselves; none of their pursuits were propelled by anonymity. Yet their enthusiasms were ultimately provoked by a humbler, profounder, and more universal story, the victim's. Consumption might strike anyone, rich or poor, oppressed or exalted. To hear the diagnosis was a confrontation with mortality. The stages and treatment of the disease became an elaborate ritual; entering a sanatorium, for example, subjected the patient to a therapeutic program long since vanished from the arsenal of medicine. This too is a story, the more worth retelling because it's beginning to be lost: few patients wrote of themselves for the general public during the great days of the sanatorium movement, and every year fewer survive to recall it.

I am interested in all these stories for their own sakes, and for the ways they intertwine. In the following pages I will be

4

exploring them all for recurring patterns and hidden themes; for the metaphors of sickness and health they generated; for what, implicitly, they may tell us about the diseases, like cancer and AIDS, that traumatize us today.

Of course, we are naturally most interested in our own human stake in any discussion of illness. But there is another, more primitive story upon which the drama of tuberculosis rests, and since it underlies so much of what will follow, perhaps we should tell it now. For, plague to humanity though it was and is, tuberculosis is also, and most basically, the life story of a microscopic curved or rod-shaped plant. It is tiny; laid end to end, it would take as many as twenty-five thousand of them to extend an inch. *Mycobacterium tuberculosis humanis,* as the organism is formally called, belongs to a large family of bacteria, only one other genus of which causes human disease (that too a dreaded one—leprosy). The *mycobacterium tuberculosis,* or tubercle bacillus, is, for a bacterium, distinctive in its habits. It needs oxygen to survive and will perish rapidly without it, no small irony considering that, in the late nineteenth century, fresh air was thought the most reliable combatant against the disease. It grows best in darkness and in moist places but can survive for up to two hours in direct sunlight, for a full day in human sputum, or for six to eight months in dried sputum kept away from sunlight. Bacilli have been stored for as long as twelve years to emerge living and virulent. For a microorganism, it reproduces slowly, doubling its numbers only once within fifteen to twenty-four hours. But that sluggish pace, laid against the far slower human life cycle, becomes frightening: a single organism will, within a few weeks, have replicated itself hundreds of millions of times. Within a month its spawn will number in the billions, swamping its host's defenses.

Yet not all tubercle bacilli cause disease. There are harmless as well as virulent strains, and the two are virtually indistinguishable from each other in appearance and biological characteristics. The only sure way to tell whether the strain in question is pathogenic is to inject it into a test animal to see if the disease develops. Alternatively, but less surely, you can simply culture the organisms. Nonvirulent strains grow patternlessly, forming, within a few days, a random heap in the culture medium. But the disease-producing strains are more deliberate, almost military: they often form serpentine cords, arranged in rough parallel. They also tend individually to be longer and more often curved than the nonvirulent strains.

However these pathogenic organisms travel—on dust particles, some scientists suppose; on airborne droplets, still more assert—as recently as fifty years ago they found their way into the bodies of as many as 90 percent of the adult population of the United States. Few of these people ever came down with a clinical case of the disease; they had merely been exposed to an infection that, thanks to vigor or luck, they managed to fight off. Tuberculosis is a highly contagious disease—it remains to this day the world's most serious bacteria-borne illness—but also one that the majority of its potential victims can effectively resist. Even in the United States today, with tuberculosis much reduced in frequency, 15 percent of adults test positively as having been exposed.

In these cases the victim apparently inhales a droplet of liquid or mote of dust, bearing a few virulent tubercle bacilli. (A larger grain, or one more heavily populated by microorganisms, would be caught and destroyed by defensive mechanisms in the nasal passages or the upper respiratory tract.) The organisms don't survive well in the larger air passages, but if they succeed in entering an alveolus (one of the minute air sacs in the lung) they have reached an ideal breeding ground.

But the body's defenses recognize the alien bacilli as a threat. As soon as they reach an alveolar space they are devoured by white blood cells, which, if previously activated by the complex workings of the body's immune system, destroy the invaders at once. Yet if a white blood cell, newly arrived in the lung, has not been sensitized, it merely engulfs the bacilli without killing them. Meant to be their destroyer, it becomes their protector; unrecognized by other components of the immune system, the bacilli multiply unmolested within the white blood cell. In this sense, although tuberculosis is often called an affliction of the lungs, it is most fundamentally a disease of the blood in general, and of white blood cells in particular.

Within a few weeks, the tubercle bacilli have spread, first to the lymph nodes nearest the site of original infection, then into the bloodstream, then everywhere. At this stage, the body, not alerted to the foreignness of the invading microbes, does not systematically attack them or endeavor to wall them off. In some organs—the liver, the bone marrow, the spleen, the lymph nodes—they are quickly killed, but in others they multiply, most often and most successfully in the apices of the lungs, where the oxygen they need to flourish and reproduce is most plentiful. But they can thrive as well in other organs: the kidneys, the ends of the long bones, and the brain.

Soon, however, the body becomes sensitized and begins actively to fight the disease. The white blood cells, now recognizing the tubercle bacilli as alien, ingest and kill them. Wherever they appear, tubercles form—small pockets with walls made of several kinds of blood cells, surrounding the bacilli. Dying, these protecting cells sometimes become soft and cheeselike in consistency; sometimes they calcify. At this point, while the tubercles are usually still too small to be seen in an X ray, the body has in fact become hypersensitive to both the bacillus and its by-products. If tuberculin, a broth made of tubercle bacilli boiled in a glycerine solution, is injected under the skin at this juncture, within a few days the skin will become inflamed, demonstrating both the presence of the germs in the body and the arousal, albeit belated, of its defenses against them.

About 85 to 90 percent of the time, the disease ends here and the bacilli spread no farther. If any remain alive, they are dormant, sealed off within the tubercles, potentially lethal but quiescent. But in the other 10 to 15 percent of cases, the disease goes on without interruption to assume its clinical form. And among the 85 to 90 percent who recover initially, about one in twenty will, later in life—either because their initially latent infections reactivate, or because of other factors, still unknown—acquire the disease in full-fledged form.

When tuberculosis, under whatever circumstances, progresses beyond this relatively harmless stage, the bacilli continue to multiply. Small patches of pneumonia may develop in the tubercles, which liquefy and empty into adjacent tissues. In the process many bacilli die, but a few survive and spread the infection still farther.

The lung (or whatever other organ is affected) appears, in other words, to be consuming itself from within, slowly in those sections relatively poor in oxygen, more rapidly elsewhere. Eventually the lesions, growing and multiplying, break out of the alveoli and empty into the bronchi, the branching air passages that penetrate the lung, whence infection can be exhaled or spat into the air and spread to others. As the liquefied dead tissue and living bacilli spill into the host's air passages, they leave behind them cavities in the lung, which afford still better breeding for the bacilli, and which have been found to harbor as many as ten billion of them.

As the lung gradually dissolves, emptying itself into the air, symptoms begin to occur. The patient coughs, first intermittently then constantly, and each spasm pushes the liquefied lung through its own air passages and out into the atmosphere. Eventually small blood vessels erode, rupture, and bleed into the sputum, which begins to be streaked with blood or becomes pinkish in color. Full-fledged hemorrhages can now occur, the patient coughing up pure blood, bright red and foamy. A daily fever appears, rising during the afternoon, then falling again at night and producing profuse night sweats. The patient begins to lose weight, tires easily, and may experience heart palpitations or chest pain as the pleura (the membrane surrounding the lungs and lining the wall of the chest cavity) becomes involved.

Though it most commonly affects the lungs because they afford it such favorable conditions, tuberculosis can spread anywhere. If it passes into the bloodstream or the lymphatic system, it can spawn innumerable tiny seedlike pods of infection throughout the body, in which case it is called miliary tuberculosis—the most rapidly and frequently fatal form of the disease. It can affect the pericardium, the membrane surrounding the heart, and can invade the stomach and the intestines, the bones and the joints, the genitals and the urinary tract.

Eventually, if it remains untreated, the patient dies, most commonly of inanition, though he can also smother, drowning in his own body fluids as they flood his destroyed lungs, or succumb when any other vital organ attacked by the disease is overwhelmed by it.

Small wonder tuberculosis has inspired a peculiar terror, and an immemorial one. For it has been known since ancient times. Traces of it have been found in Egyptian skeletons dating from 3700 B.C.; there is some evidence that a special hospital for the tubercular existed as early as 1000 B.C. But like most diseases, consumption (or phthisis, as its pulmonary version is often called) has ebbed and flowed, not afflicting all times and places equally.

Contagious illnesses typically follow an epidemic curve, at first rising rapidly in frequency, reaching a plateau, then gradually subsiding. Tuberculosis is no exception, but its cycles are apparently unusually slow, not spanning months or decades but centuries: at present we are living at the apparent end of a long epidemic wave, which appears to have begun in Europe in the late seventeenth century, just as the industrial revolution commenced, as towns began to turn from overgrown villages into sprawling metropolises, as science came of age and the pace of its discoveries began to accelerate. It is, historically, coeval with the emergence of the modern world, and an affliction that its students often identified with the complexity and stress of modern urban living. By the mid-nineteenth century, when mortality from tuberculosis reached its peak, it had claimed millions, if not tens of millions. At the end of the 1800s it still killed a seventh of the human race, and as late as the 1940s it continued to cause more deaths than any other contagious disease. And it was an indiscriminate, universal, and democratic leveler. The poor, packed into tenements, were particularly susceptible, but the rich and eminent were not exempt. Poe, Lanier, Chopin, Stevenson, Napoleon, Emerson, Keats—all either had it or thought they did. Consumption stalked the cities, but the countryside fell victim as well. It throve in the smoke and dust of sweatshops, but it also prospered in the sealed and overheated parlors of the bourgeoisie. It was no respecter of age, sex, or occupation, and by the 1870s, it had been so effectively publicized as widespread, invidious, and invariably fatal that it had come, in the popular imagination, nearly to stand for death itself.

Over the course of centuries, treatments for the disease changed with the fashions of medicine. Every imaginable theory had its airing. In imperial Rome, consumptives were typically sent to warm, dry climates. Claudius Galenus (A.D. 130?–201?), the legendary Greek authority, prescribed rest, residence underground, and fresh milk (woman's, camel's, ass's, and goat's). Some authorities advised inactivity, others exercise, especially on horseback. (Thomas Sydenham, the great seventeenth-century English physician, was a particularly influential proponent of the latter activity.) Sea air, seaweed, mountain air, cold air, warm air, sunlight—all had advocates. Sidney Lanier went to Florida in search of health; Robert Louis Stevenson from Scotland to the Adirondacks to Tahiti. Folklore prescribed various nostra—Pliny suggested a wolf's liver boiled in wine. Benevolent deities and patron saints might be invoked; and as the industrial revolution spread, patent medicines began to be offered to the public, and specifics hopefully prescribed. For a time arsenic found partisans; so did creosote, gold, and copper salts. Even pioneers of the antituberculosis movement tried some therapies that seem bizarre by modern standards—hydrogen sulfide gas and medicated oxygen inhaled as the patient sat in a glass cabinet. At the turn of the century one could buy various antitubercular concoctions at the neighborhood drugstore: Piso's Cure for Consumption, Schenck's Pulmonic Syrup, Helmbold's Buchu Extract.

Remedies, until the nineteenth century, were far more easily available than fundamental facts about the disease. Only by the mid-nineteenth century had enough accurate information been amassed to allow for a thorough description of the disease process in the lungs and in other affected tissues. Not until 1865 was it proved to be contagious; not until 1882 did Robert Koch, working in Berlin, finally isolate the tubercle bacillus, describe it, and convict it of causing pulmonary consumption. It was a quantum leap in knowledge, but of ambiguous benefit, since it proved frustratingly slow in producing effective therapies. The microscope, as little by little it revealed the habits of the microbe, explained why traditional remedies didn't work, but failed for decades to identify one that would.

Still, as the nineteenth century drew to a close, more and more scientists and physicians drew together in a consensus about how best to contain the disease, if not absolutely to cure it: bacteriological discoveries had not yielded a foolproof weapon against tuberculosis, but they had suggested a reasonable strategy for retarding its spread. First, since it was now known to be contagious and the mechanism of infection understood, it made sense as far as possible to isolate the tubercular, under conditions as pleasant as possible, from the general population. And further, it came to be thought that the tubercles, the destructive consequences of the illness, might be used to frustrate it. If the lungs were made as inactive as possible, the walls of the tubercles, gradually thickening and strengthening, might seal the bacilli off, protecting the surrounding tissue from infection. The disease, not strictly speaking cured, would at least subside into quiescence; gradually and carefully, by graded stages, the patient might resume activity, eventually returning as an arrested case to normal life.

This theory—and even now opinion remains divided as to whether or not it worked, and exactly how it worked if in fact it did—gave rise to the rest cure, the sanatorium culture immortalized by Thomas Mann in *The Magic Mountain* and elsewhere. Until the discovery of antibiotics, it dominated the treatment of tuberculosis, at least in orthodox medical circles, and it took two forms, the first institutional, the second surgical.

In Europe and America, Gustav Herrmann Brehmer, Peter Dettweiler, and Edward Livingston Trudeau pioneered the

sanatorium rest routine, sequestering their patients in sprawling rural hospitals, isolated from the great centers of population. Patients at these institutions followed varying routines
and underwent different treatments, but, eventually, whatever else they did, they rested; reading, sleeping, looking out
at the spectacular scenery sanatoriums usually tried to furnish,
hoping to while away consumption, allowing their bodies to
spin the delicate threads of tissue that would contain the disease. But in Italy, in 1892, Carlo Forlanini devised a more
invasive method for inducing the lung to rest. If nitrogen was
injected between the ribs into the chest cavity, the lung would
collapse, rendered temporarily inactive. The healing would
thus proceed uninterrupted while the remaining lung carried
on the work of respiration. Artificial pneumothorax, as this
procedure was called, won an official endorsement from the
International Congress of Tuberculosis at Rome in 1912 and
thereafter joined the rest cure to become a frequent fixture of
a sanatorium stay during the 1920s and 1930s. Where, for one
reason or another, pneumothorax failed to produce an effective collapse, other surgical treatments might be tried, more
radical and more traumatic, but reputedly more effective.

In some, if not all cases the sanatorium routine and collapse
therapy worked, either separately or together. Mortality from
tuberculosis, gradually falling ever since the middle of the
nineteenth century, began to plunge more steeply; between
1904, the year the National Association for the Study and Prevention of Tuberculosis was founded, and 1919, the death rate
fell 33 percent; it plummeted from 188.1 per 100,000 in 1904
to 40.1 per 100,000 in 1945.

Despite these apparently dramatic advances, there remained the persistent desire for a specific cure. Penicillin had
first been identified in 1929 and had proved effective against
cocci and certain other bacteria, but not the tubercle bacillus,
which carries a waxy coating impervious to it. Neither it nor
the sulfa drugs, despite early hopes, afforded the answer. But,
beginning in the 1930s, new experimental evidence began to
emerge; *mycobacterium tuberculosis humanis* began to show

some vulnerabilities. It was found that certain fungi were able to repress its development and that, though it multiplies freely in *sterile* soil, something in fresh, unsterilized dirt retarded its ability to reproduce. And some protozoa were found that, despite the tubercle bacillus's normal indigestibility, were able to engulf it.

There the matter remained, however, until the early 1940s, when a New Jersey farmer, troubled by a persistent infection among his chickens (which they appeared to be gobbling up from the dirt in their barnyard), brought them to a microbiology laboratory at Rutgers University, where they were examined by the late Selman Waksman, his colleagues, and students. The soil the chickens were swallowing proved to harbor a fungus that, apart from its ability to cause infection on its own, turned out as well to produce a bacteriostatic substance, which, after refinement and experiment, came to be called streptomycin.

It was first tried on tuberculosis patients at the Mayo Clinic in the winter of 1944–45. Despite some undesirable side effects, patients treated with it showed marked and startling improvements. Within weeks, tubercle bacilli vanished from their sputum, a process that the rest cure took at best months or years to complete. Symptoms cleared and did not return; patients who had entered the hospital with the gloomy prospect of years of inactivity before them were able in some cases to return to home and work almost immediately. And streptomycin opened a floodgate; within a few years an armamentarium of other effective drugs emerged, culminating in 1951 with the most powerful of all, isoniazid. Isoniazid had been known since 1912, ironically, just when scientists began to envision and experiment with naturally-occurring bacteriostatic substances, but had never before been used as an antibiotic or tried on tuberculosis. Tested in the wake of streptomycin's success, it proved more effective while producing fewer side effects. It works relatively slowly, like all the antituberculosis drugs: they retard the microbe's growth rather than killing it outright, and hence operate only when the bacterium is active and metabolizing. They have no effect during the frequent intervals when the germs are dormant, so the treatment must be continued over an extended period, and is most effective when it includes a combination of drugs. But the results are immediate and dramatic. Within three months of their first treatment, 90 percent of patients show no sign of infection; *mycobacterium tuberculosis* can no longer be cultured from them.

Thus, in the 1950s the solemn shadow of the White Plague vanished with a suddenness that quite literally left the tubercular dancing in the aisles of their sanatoriums (though that was largely inspired by one experimental antibiotic, iproniazid, which proved to have a marked euphoric as well as a bacteriostatic effect, and was quickly withdrawn). Consumption shrank to a condition requiring a short stint on bed rest followed by a year or two of pill taking. Sanatoriums languished as their patients went home, finding themselves refuges for the generally decrepit rather than for the tubercular; only those too old to readjust to normal life or too debilitated from other conditions remained. Pneumothorax disappeared from medical textbooks as a surgical technique, remaining only as the description of what happened after an accidental puncture of the chest cavity. In 1954 the trustees of the Trudeau Sanatorium in Saranac Lake decided to close the nation's pioneer tuberculosis hospital; others followed soon after. By 1960 the sanatorium had largely disappeared from the American landscape, to become a memory among its ex-patients, an outmoded and forgotten byway in medical history. The buildings became schools, nursing homes, or prisons (minimum security, mostly). The National Tuberculosis Association (which had begun in 1904 as the National Association for the Study and Prevention of Tuberculosis, then shortened its name) became the American Lung Association, turning its formidable powers of publicity to a campaign against smoking.

A few sanatoriums struggled along into the early 1970s. Their patients and staff, grown used to their routine, clung to it: when New York closed its last state hospital, the Homer

Folks Sanatorium in Oneonta, it encountered some difficulty dislodging the supervising physician from his official residence, even though the hospital was empty, its patients all gone home, and the rest of the staff departed for other jobs. Alumni of the sanatoriums even now remember their experiences not with the distaste one might expect, but with nostalgia, fondness, and even a regret as for something lost.

The War on Consumption, and the sanatorium culture it spawned, were together a way of life for five generations of Americans, well and ill. We may think of them as unfortunate, haunted by a plague destined to vanish overnight, but they did not think of themselves that way. Their story is a fragment of American history, misplaced and in danger of being lost. Reconstructing it will, I hope, teach us something about health, something about mortality, and something about the ways, perforce or by choice, we adjust to both.

1

"*The Sorrow of the Cities*":
Images of Tuberculosis in the Nineteenth Century

The sorrow of the cities, the dark curse
Of toil that buys but toil and poverty,
Plagues bred in crowded alleys, ignorance
Of the wise, gold-lust, neglect, the love
Unschooled to guard its own, have made
These little threads so weak and delicate
That they are scarcely twilled before they break.
—THE GODDESS HYGEIA, IN
"THE NARROW DOOR" (1915)

In the spring of 1862, Henry David Thoreau was dying. The fierce individualist, intrepid naturalist, resourceful *bricoleur* who had lived a year on the shore of Walden Pond in a shack of his own making, now lay at the age of forty-five, helpless on a rattan daybed in the parlor of his parents' prim home on Main Street in Concord. The once-rugged outdoorsman, as his lungs gave out and his strength ebbed, found himself surrounded by pale, polite Concord ladies—his mother, his Aunt Louisa (who solemnly asked, had he made his peace with God?), and his maiden sister Sophia, who helped him beguile wakeful nights by rearranging the parlor furniture in the firelight to make it cast fantastic shadows on the wall. The renegade who had spent a night in the town jail, cellmate to an accused barnburner, now received sentimental visits from his jailer ("Never spent an hour with more satisfaction," Thoreau afterward told Ralph Waldo Emerson); Judge Hoar sent hyacinths; another friend, some homemade jelly.

Thoreau had been struck by consumption, the plague that in the mid-nineteenth century carried off more Americans than any other disease; to contract it, conventional wisdom ran, meant a slow and a certain, but also a dignified, even a radiant death. In 1862 there was no selfish dread, no panic among his Concord neighbors and friends, for consumption, though thought of as inevitably fatal, was not widely believed to be contagious. So instead of acute terror, it aroused a pleasing melancholy, even a pious exhilaration. In fact, during the earlier decades of the nineteenth century, of all diseases tuberculosis had a reputation more calculated to draw admiration than repulsion, particularly in transcendentalist Concord. For among illnesses, tuberculosis was seen as the most spiritual, the most ennobling, a purger of base qualities and a distiller of lofty ones. Popular opinion ignored, or at least minimized, the often hideous physical symptoms—none of Thoreau's intimates, at least in the written record of his last months, chose to remark upon the horror of seeing a once-robust man who had earned his keep as a day laborer reduced to a wraith, scarcely able to lift a pencil and dependent on an amanuensis for drafting even a short letter.

Instead, they saw what generations had chosen to see since the late seventeenth century, when consumption had begun to emerge as a major factor in European mortality. It was, Sir Thomas Browne wrote in 1657, "one of the mercifullest executives of death, whose blows are scarce to be felt, which no man would be killed to be free of, wherein a man is led, not torn, unto his transition, may number his days and even his last hours and speak unto his savior when he is within a moment of him." As the victim passed through the stages of the illness, the encumbering accretions of his personality melted away, revealing the spiritual matrices out of which the transitory and illusory accidents of his character had been formed.

No one illustrates better than Thoreau the degree to which this myth of the disease could overshadow reality. Thoreau was, on the face of it, an unlikely candidate for etherealization. In fact he was stubborn, craggy, temperamental, as much in character heaving manure as spinning theories. It was probably he who invented a manufacturing process that turned the

17

family pencil-making business from a hand-to-mouth venture into a consistently profitable operation. And he had always been practical about money; even on his deathbed he was not solely engaged in contemplating the transcendent: his last letter was to James T. Fields, the editor of the *Atlantic Monthly*:

> Only extreme illness has prevented my answering your note earlier. I have no objection to having the papers you refer to printed in your monthly—if my feeble health will permit me to prepare them for the printer. What will you give me for them?

He had scandalized Concord in 1844 by starting a forest fire along the Sudbury River ("a damned rascal," the fire fighters had called him; "Burnt woods!" the townspeople used to shout after him as he sauntered down the street). "I have never been able to understand what he meant by his life," wrote his close friend William Ellery Channing, "why he was so disappointed with everybody else &c. Why was he so much interested in the river and the woods and the sky &c. Something peculiar I judge."

But now that he lay moribund, Concord and consumption worked together to spiritualize him. "He died of consumption. His was a tranquil death, an euthanasia befitting such an exalted spirit," according to a contemporary obituary. "In the prime of his power . . . [he] passed away from the sensible world, called Nature, which he enjoyed so keenly and understood so well, into that spiritual sphere of which Nature is a mere symbol and changing shadow." Sophia wrote in the same vein to a friend, who, perhaps a little ghoulishly, asked for an account of Henry's last illness and death:

> I feel like saying that Henry was never affected, never reached by it. I never before saw such a manifestation of the power of spirit over matter. Very often I have heard him tell his visitors that he enjoyed existence as well as ever. He remarked to me that there was as much comfort in perfect disease as in perfect health, the mind always conforming to the condition of the body. The thought of

death, he said, could not begin to trouble him. His thoughts entertained him all his life, and did still.

The Concord schoolchildren were given a holiday for his funeral and marched before the procession, throwing wild-flowers in its path. There were Bible readings and a plaintive funeral ode read by Channing, but the occasion gained a lasting symbolic stamp only from Emerson's funeral address, which was later printed in the *Atlantic*. Perhaps more than any other single influence, it helped perpetuate the myth of Thoreau as an ascetic, a renouncer of the surfaces of nature and a seeker of the transcendent. Cranky acts of will, bending before the power of Emersonian rhetoric, became triumphs of self-denial: "Few lives contain so many renunciations. He was bred to no profession; he never married; he lived alone; he never went to church; he never voted; he refused to pay a tax to the state; he ate no flesh, he drank no wine, he never knew the use of tobacco." His skirmishes with Concord and his refusal to join its currents were spiritual manifestations; his final illness, instead of an untimely and ironic blow of fate, became the expression of a delicacy too pure for life; his death the inevitable consequence of a perilous quest for the spirit:

There is a flower known to botanists, one of the same genus with our summer plant called "Life-Everlasting," a *Graphalium* like that, which grows on the most inaccessible cliffs of the Tyrolean mountains, where the chamois dare hardly venture, and which the hunter, tempted by its beauty, and by his love (for it is immensely valued by the Swiss maidens), climbs the cliffs to gather, and is sometimes found dead at the feet, with the flower in his hand. It is called by . . . the Swiss *Edelweisse*, which signifies *Noble Purity*. Thoreau seemed to me living in the hope to gather this plant, which belonged to him of right. . . . Wherever there is knowledge, wherever there is virtue, wherever there is beauty, he will find a home.

The impulse to transform this intransigent eccentric into a messenger of the spirit gained something from Emerson and

Concord transcendentalism, but it was also rooted firmly in contemporary beliefs about consumption. It was a gentle death, the soft peril of those who scorned attachment to the solidity of matter. It was a badge of refinement, it was very nearly a polite accomplishment. And if you contracted it, it led your friends not to mourn your early death so much as to venerate you as one marked out for a fate of special distinction.

That made a certain amount of sense. The symptoms of the disease—a gradual loss of flesh, the sparkling eyes, the flush and slight excitement brought on by low-grade fever—all these suggested immateriality, a looking toward the beyond. And somehow these symptoms outweighed the more frightening and disgusting ones. Sidney Lanier, another American literary figure afflicted with tuberculosis and fated to die of it at the dawn of the sanatorium era in 1881, never minimized the agony his condition caused. In a letter to his brother, he described his debilitating and implacable fever as "most peculiar and baffling. I cannot locate it in any limb or organ, just as one cannot locate thirst, which is a lack in the whole blood; a severe fever comes—or rather stays, it never goes—and therewith a general discomfort under which I can scarcely refrain from such groans and shrieks as a wounded dog gives, crawling off with a broken back and hind-legs dragging." Yet in December of 1880 he wrote, while running a fever of 104 degrees, one of his best-known poems, "Sunrise," and insofar as it can be read as a covert commentary on his illness, it conforms to the conventional view of the disease as an ennobling and spiritual-izing force.

The narrator, dreaming in a restless sleep of "the live-oak, the marsh, and the main," awakes and goes out, mesmerically drawn to the littoral marsh that is the chief symbolic presence in the poem:

> Reverend Marsh, low-couched along the sea,
>   Old chemist, rapt in alchymy,
>   Distilling silence,—lo,
> That which our father-age had died to know—
> The menstruum that dissolves all matter—thou

Hast found it: for this silence, filling now
The globed clarity of receiving space,
This solves us all: man, matter, doubt, disgrace,
    Death, love, sin, sanity.

In the marsh, as in the physical distress of the disease, everything softens, decays, and degenerates into a great primal ra-
gout. Hard-edged distinctions are lost, and everything blends;
the very vagueness and dissolution of the landscape, however,
renders it a fitter setting for the sunrise that comprises the
poem's spectacular conclusion. It, plainly, represents the triumph of spirit, rising out of the decay and made more spectacularly clear by the contrast with it. One's separate being
must be rendered, rotted—in short, consumed—before one
can properly behold the splendor of the light.

How dark, how dark soever the race that
    must needs be run,
      I am lit with the Sun . . .
And even my heart through the night shall
    with knowledge abide thee,
And ever by day shall my spirit, as one
    that hath tried thee
Labor, at leisure, in art—till yonder
    beside thee
      My soul shall float, friend Sun,
        The day being done.

The Latin root of the most common nineteenth-century word
for the disease, "consumption," echoes Lanier's conceit: *con*
(meaning "completely"), plus *sumere*, "to take up from under"
or "to buy." The body, this etymology suggests, is not merely
being wasted or squandered, but being taken *up*, raised,
bought. By what, then, if not the spirit? Remember, the tubercle bacillus was not discovered until 1882, and when Robert
Koch announced his epoch-making find, he was met in the
nonscientific press with a combination of indifference and
skepticism. The public were most dubious about the existence
of marauding germs and did not widely accept the image of a

body being gobbled up by microscopic gluttons; they could not easily visualize anything doing the consuming. The most widely held belief, among doctors as well as laymen, was that the disease might be provoked by the environment, but that most fundamentally it was a manifestation of the victim's own constitution. And if that constitution chose to devour the very body in which it resided, what better proof of its dedication to the immaterial?

Even the purely economic meaning we now mostly ascribe to "consumption" has roots surprisingly connected to this idea. Thorstein Veblen devised his theory of conspicuous consumption precisely at the height of the American war on tuberculosis. His idea, simply put, was that early in the history of human society, the unproductive consumption of goods became a mark of honor and dignity. Acquiring useless, or even harmful things like alcohol, unhealthy foods, impractical clothes, was seen as a sign of one's liberation from the yokes of labor and necessity; it showed how far one had advanced past the point where one's whole time and substance were taken up in acquiring the necessities of living.

If a wasteful consumption of food, drink, and fancy goods is proof of nobility and refinement, how much greater a leap in distinction must it not be if one can similarly waste one's own body? To do so places one not merely at the top of social and economic hierarchies but also atop a spiritual one. The act of consumption is more conspicuous if it makes a deliberately pointless use of something necessary in another context: Veblen traces, for example, the fashion for smooth green lawns back to an earlier cattle-raising culture. Clipped turf flaunts the owner's freedom from a need to use his land for grazing, and reminds the viewer how far he is above crass economic imperatives. And if, through an impulse of your constitution, you contract a disease that consumes your body, you are demonstrating how much more triumphant is your conquest of the flesh than humanity's at large: mankind's most basic necessity is your expendable luxury.

In nineteenth-century literature, this is the role the consumptive most typically assumes. The Goncourt brothers, in *Madame Gervaisais,* offered this as an objective account:

> In contrast to the diseases of the crude, baser organs of the body which clog and soil the mind, the imagination, and the very humors of the sick as though with corrupt matter, phthisis, this illness of the lofty and noble parts of the human being, calls forth in the patient a state of elevation, tenderness and love, a new urge to see the good, the beautiful and the ideal in everything, a state of human sublimity which seems almost not to be of this earth.

Even while such descriptions as this were being written, pathologists were discovering and describing the soggy mess tuberculosis actually made of the lungs, the massive corruption it left in its wake. But scientific discovery penetrated the medical profession at a slow pace, and the general public at a glacial one. Old images persisted hardily against new information; physicians themselves, long after the facts might have persuaded them otherwise, continued to picture their consumptive patients in the old way. In an 1830 issue of *Blackwoods Magazine,* in an article entitled, "Affecting Scenes: Passages from the Diary of a Physician," a doctor described the case of "Little Eliza Herbert":

> Little Eliza had inherited, with her mother's beauty, her constitutional delicacy. Her figure was so slight, that it almost suggested to the beholder the idea of transparency; and there was a softness and languor in her azure eyes beaming through their long silken lashes, which told of something too refined for humanity.

After being dispatched—futilely, as it turns out—to Italy, Eliza returns home and expires luminously:

> She was wasted almost to a shadow,—attenuated to nearly ethereal delicacy and transparency. . . . Perfectly motionless and statuelike lay that fair creature, breathing so imperceptibly that a rose-leaf might have slept on her lips unfluttered.

Whether Little Eliza was a real case history or a figure of her chronicler's imagination, she is not alone in early-nineteenth-century accounts of the disease, whether fictional, nominally factual, or actually factual. The note recurs in dozens of tuber-cular and crypto-tubercular deaths. Paul Dombey is a notable example in Charles Dickens's *Dombey and Son;* so is Beth in Louisa May Alcott's *Little Women.*

> When Jo came home that spring, she had been struck with the change in Beth. No one spoke of it or seemed aware of it, for it had come too gradually to startle those who saw her daily; but to eyes sharpened by absence it was very plain, and a heavy weight fell on Jo's heart as she saw her sister's face. It was no paler, and but little thinner than in autumn; yet there was a strange transparent look about it, as if the mortal was being slowly refined away, and the immortal shining through the frail flesh with an indescrib-ably pathetic beauty.

When Beth's end comes, it descends on her with the gentle-ness supposed typical of the disease: "in the dark hour before the dawn, on the bosom where she had drawn her first breath, she quietly drew her last, with no farewell but one loving look and a little sigh."

Descriptions of the expiring consumptive often evince an unsettling satisfaction, as if the invalid's death were not merely edifying to the observer, or even an occasion for self-satisfac-tion in the survivor, but an erotic *frisson.* The spectacle of the victim revealing more and more of herself through ever more diaphanous veils of flesh arouses the keeper of the bedside vigil, even as the consumptive's increasing weakness and pas-sivity put her more and more within his power. Supine, per-haps, she is no longer potentially a demanding partner; weak-ness has rendered her safe for the observer's imagination. The note is struck clearly in the passage on Little Eliza Herbert, but the fervor of the langauge implies it even in Alcott.

In a cultural milieu where sex was little written about, it was no great leap from the idealistic to the erotic; the former could, apparently innocently, garb itself in the ardor of the latter, the writer remaining entirely unconscious of the subtext. One could talk freely, even passionately, about consumption, because it was so inward, spiritual, and ennobling. Little wonder that darker and more unruly forces—Mors and Eros—should roost on it, and the transparency of the consumptive reveal truths more unsettling than reassuring. This is nowhere clearer than in the greatest, the most influential, and the most conscious of all the consumption novels, Alexandre Dumas fils' *The Lady of the Camellias.* Both the book and its enormously successful stage version contributed to the myth of tuberculosis as a spiritualizing force: what more powerful argument than the worldly courtesan turned to courses of self-denial and sacrifice by the combined power of her advancing disease and her ennobling passion for Armand Duval?

Dumas milks that theme expertly, but mingles it as well with darker undercurrents. The novel opens with a striking tableau: the narrator visits a display and auction of the late courtesan's personal effects. Marguerite's death reveals the secrets of her life as nothing in the life itself could or would:

> I discovered without difficulty that I was in the house of a kept woman. . . . This one was dead, so the most virtuous of women could enter even her bedroom. Death had purified the air of this abode of splendid foulness, and if more excuse were needed, they had the excuse that they had merely come to a sale, they knew not whose.

Her illness and death have burnt away her notoriety and rendered her goods fit prey for another kind of consumption, a buying spree by the Paris *bourgeoises.* But her death also makes for another and much more horrifying epiphany. Returning after her burial, and having learned the unselfish reasons for which she deserted him, Armand insists on having the body exhumed at Père Lachaise for a final look. When Marguerite's face is revealed, what her lover sees colors all the rest of the story and casts a pall on any easy assumptions we might make as to the nobility of tuberculosis—Armand sees a parody of consumptive transparency, an extension of its proverbial revelation of the spirit into a revelation of death and decay.

> It was terrible to see, it is horrible to relate. The eyes were nothing but two holes, the lips had disappeared, vanished, and the white teeth were tightly set. The black hair, long and dry, was pressed tightly about the forehead, and half veiled the green hollows of the cheeks; and yet I recognized in this face the joyous white and rose face that I had seen so often.

Armand, unable to turn away his eyes, puts his handkerchief to his mouth and bites it.

As a fitting memorial, a tribute to Marguerite's nobility, and a reminder of their love, Armand arranges for fresh camellias always to be placed on her grave. They are indeed a memento, but more as well—they are the badge of her sexuality, explicit enough to have caused more than one Victorian controversy. At the beginning of the novel the narrator disingenuously pretends puzzlement at the meaning of Marguerite's habit of wearing white camellias twenty-five days of every month and red ones for the remaining five. But any doubts are resolved by Armand in his description of their mutual seduction, which begins, significantly, with a tubercular hemorrhage:

> The room to which she had fled was lit only by a single candle. She lay back on a great sofa, her dress undone, holding one hand on her heart, and letting the other hang by her side. On the table was a basin half full of water, and the water was stained with streaks of blood.

The grisly sight, however, leads to an assignation, upon the completion of which Marguerite announces why she can't perform on her promise at once:

> "If I decide now on taking a new lover, he must have three very rare qualities: he must be confiding, submissive, and discreet."
> "Well, I will be all that you wish."
> "We shall see."
> "When shall we see?"
> "Later on."

"Why?"

"Because," said Marguerite, releasing herself from my arms, and, taking from a great bunch of red camellias a single camellia, she placed it in my buttonhole, "because one can not always carry out agreements the day they are signed."

"And when shall I see you again?" I said, clasping her in my arms.

"When this camellia changes color."

The blood of the tubercular hemorrhage blends metaphorically with menstrual blood. Both are signs of mixed uncleanness and attraction; sickness and death blend inextricably with sexuality and procreation.

Marguerite goes on, in the course of the novel, to ennoble herself immensely, unselfishly renouncing Armand at his father's bidding in order to protect his inheritance. The increasing vulnerability her illness imposes on her makes her all the more selfless, without, however, making her any the less voluptuous. Dumas was either bold or oblivious enough to bring all these themes together, at the brink of explicitness and occasionally over it. But he was not alone: the Henri Murger story on which *La Bohème* is based, "Francine and Her Muff," similarly mixes spirituality, eroticism, and death in the crucible of consumption, evoking Dionysiac themes that Puccini still less allowed in his opera than Verdi had in *La Traviata*.

Francine, the original of Mimi, initiates an affair with Jacques (the prototype for Rodolfo): "She had known nothing about love till she was over twenty, but a vague presentiment of her early death warned her not to delay too much if she ever wanted to know what love was." They both embark on their relation knowing Francine has consumption, romantically sensing that their summer burns the more brightly for the imminence of Francine's certain doom. "Bother the dead leaves," she tells Jacques. "Never mind about the autumn; it is summer now, and the leaves are still green. Let us make the most of it, my dear. When you see that I am going to leave you, you shall take me in your arms and kiss me and tell me to stay. You know how obedient I am, and stay I will."

27

She expires, picturesquely, with the last dead leaf, heightened both sexually and ethically. Like Armand, Jacques can't leave his dead mistress alone, as if mortality had all along been part of her fascination. He has a postmortem cast made of her head, and the process triggers an epiphany less grisly than Marguerite Gauthier's, but composed of the same elements.

> Now a strange thing happened. A change took place in Francine's face. The blood, which had not had time to become quite cold, possibly warmed by the heat of the plaster, seemed to flow back again to the head, and a transparent pink flush gradually overspread the dull white of her forehead and cheeks. The eyelids, which had been raised by taking off the cast, showed the calm blue of her eyes, and there seemed a sort of intelligence in their look. A half-smile parted her lips, which seemed to be shaping the last word, forgotten in her farewell, which her lover had only heard with his heart.

For good or ill, consumption makes death into its own transfiguration, blurring the lines between eros and agape, refinement and corruption. Louisa May Alcott and Dickens were, of course, less unflinching than their French counterparts, but, though more elliptically, Paul Dombey and Beth radiate the same ambiguities.

And the note was not even entirely absent from the Concord obsequies over the dead Thoreau. The edelweiss, the flower Emerson pictured him seeking, was a token of love and an emblem of death as well as a badge of immortality. For the nineteenth-century mind, consumption was a condition in which these apparently contradictory but subliminally (and explosively) connected themes were allowed to touch. Somehow it sanitized them, legitimized them.

But new forces were at work, even as Thoreau's funeral procession made its way to the Concord graveyard. For the scientists were on the march. Philosophers fulminated and novelists imagined; but pathologists cut up cadavers and began carefully describing, for the first time, exactly what consumption did to the lungs. Where their contemporaries imagined spiritual refinement, they saw massive tissue destruction and purulence. For Little Eliza Herbert's doctor, her illness was an emanation of her own constitution, but in France in 1865, J.-A. Villemin conducted a series of experiments, at the time little publicized, that proved conclusively that tuberculosis was contagious, though he was unable to identify the medium of contagion. In 1866, scientists put sputum and lung tissue under the microscope and, for the first time, saw bacteria and spirochetes in them. By 1872, the anatomy of the tubercle had been described in detail, and several experimenters had managed to produce tuberculosis in test animals by inoculating them with infected material. Increasingly, tuberculosis began to yield to careful measurement and painstaking, hardheaded observation, and a dark though titillating myth began to give way to a mundane and ugly reality.

America lagged well behind Europe in the pace of discovery. Basic science had always suffered neglect here, obscured by the nation's infatuation with practical pursuits: engineers were far more immediately valuable than microbiologists. But even in the wake of the Civil War, and in a cultural landscape hostile or indifferent to science, new currents had begun to flow. Americans might not warm to the discoveries of cellular pathology, but they were susceptible to the proposition that tuberculosis might not be a mystic visitation but rather a practical evil, caused by clearly identifiable conditions, and therefore, perhaps, remediable. So, anyway, it seemed to Dr. Henry Bowditch of Boston, and in 1869 he published a three-article series in the *Atlantic Monthly*, "Consumption in America." The articles reflect a new spirit and amount to a fresh, pragmatic manifesto, an early messianic call for a war on tuberculosis. No longer, according to Bowditch, was a victim to bear the disease with hopeless patience, consoled only by the knowledge that his dissolution would purify him and edify his friends. Now there was hope that patience, aided by good hygiene, could actually *conquer* consumption. It might still afflict the preternaturally sensitive, but Bowditch believed they could, with proper determination, overcome it.

His shining ideals were practical and homely: good drainage, pure air, and sunlight. As a paradigm he cites two healthy brothers who marry two healthy sisters. "One lived on the old homestead, on the southern slope of one of the numerous beautiful and well-drained hills in that vicinity." But the other unwisely builds in a damp bottom.

> Through this meadow sluggishly crept the millstream of the adjacent village. Still further, all these surroundings were enclosed by lofty hills. The life-giving sun rose later and set earlier upon this than upon the other fair homestead. Till late in the forenoon, and long before sunset left the hillside home, damp and chilling emanations arose from the meadow, and day after day enveloped the tender forms of the children that were *trying in vain to grow* up healthily within them.

The valley children languish, turn consumptive, and fade away.

Disease lurks in the damp, shaded valley but can be defeated in the open air and sunlight. Though Bowditch considers the possibility that consumption is contagious, he doesn't posit a disease-carrying microbe, flourishing under the right conditions, carrying infection from one tender form to another. Instead he speaks as if sickness came *directly* from dampness, chill, and darkness. Light and air, by contrast, cure, also directly:

> It is too cold, too hot, too windy or too blustering. These and a hundred other trivial deviations from perfect weather are noted, and the unfortunate invalid quietly stays within doors day after day to avoid them. Nothing is more pernicious, no behavior more unwise. Both invalids and healthy persons ought to eschew all such views as arrant folly. "Whenever *in doubt,*" we say to our patients, "about going out, *always go out.*"

Indeed, even the cozy Victorian family circle gathered around the hearth in winter, far from a nest of well-being, is a source of disease. The sealing indoors of the family breeds consumption. Any sort of crowding, closeness, attachment is bad; freedom and space are good. Bowditch is not like his

European contemporaries, looking for answers to the scourge in a careful, methodical analysis of diseased tissue; he turns instead to the human environment. What in it was healthful, what baneful? Not surprisingly, given the post-Romantic values current in his time—and the appalling condition of its cities—space, air, sunlight, and freedom strike him as salutary; confinement and crowding, as the bearers of pestilence.

Yet, of course, they are harms that can be remedied, if only one chooses to live right, as Catherine E. Beecher and her sister-in-law Harriet Beecher Stowe maintained in their redoubtable domestic bible, *The American Woman's Home, or, Principles of Domestic Science.* The Beechers' common sense has a militant, warlike tone as suggestive of Islamic jihad as domestic science, and their call for pure air is particularly ringing.

> Little Jim, who, fresh from his afternoon's ramble in the fields, last evening said his prayers dutifully, and lay down to sleep in a most Christian frame, this morning sits up in bed with his hair bristling with crossness, strikes at his nurse, and declares he won't say his prayer's [*sic*]—that he don't want to be good. The simple difference is, that the child, having slept in a close box of a room, his brain fed all night by poison, is in a mild state of moral insanity. Delicate women remark that it takes them till eleven or twelve o'clock to get up their strength in the morning. Query, do they sleep with closed windows and doors, and with heavy bed-curtains?

Tuberculosis now begins to be spoken of as inseparable from the life being lived around it, a natural product of a bad atmosphere: the older tendency to view it as a spiritual mystery has begun to fade; the study of its sources and remedies becomes as much a branch of urban planning or domestic science as medicine. Bowditch's article, scientifically respectable though it was, owed as much in its composition to the theme of home life as to the pathology of disease. The Beechers lay out in rich detail (including even architectural drawings) their prescription for domestic happiness, title their chapter "A Christian

House," but assert that the way to achieve this is not pious meditation but know-how. The Christian housewife must design her own stove, build beds, regulate water closets, and—most vital—install an elaborate system of ventilation, instructions for which fill a whole chapter. In fact, all the progressive, forward-looking authorities had conceived, after the discovery of oxygen in the eighteenth century, a passion for "pure air," a conviction that it was necessary for health, and a strong suspicion of carbonic acid (as carbon dioxide was ominously called) as a factor in the development of consumption. In his 1872 treatise, *On the Treatment of Pulmonary Consumption by Hygiene, Climate, and Medicine,* Dr. J. H. Bennet, a Scots physician and recovered consumptive, counts tainted air as a prime cause of tuberculosis in particular and all ill-being in general: "I myself, on one occasion, became oppressed and faint when all but alone in the immense but unventilated cathedral of Milan, no doubt from the stratum of carbonic acid lying on its floor."

Consumption thus became a disease of the atmosphere; it seeped into you from the defects of your surroundings. This idea grasped the public imagination before it was proved the disease was caused by microbes, but somehow persisted, even among the scientific, long after. Sir William Osler, a patriarchal figure in scientific medicine, writing in 1892, retains his forebears' preoccupation with pure air as both a prophylactic and a curative: "The requirements of a suitable climate are a *pure atmosphere,* an *equable temperature* not subject to rapid variations, and a *maximum amount of sunshine.*" In his account of his bout with the disease, Bennet, having been diagnosed as tubercular, flees the city, its entanglements, its laden air:

> I went from Edinburgh to Loch Awe to boat and fish, whilst my friends in London were winding up my affairs. That done I departed for the Riviera . . . free from all professional ties and duties, present and future, and there settled at Mentone. For two years I entirely avoided professional occupation of any kind, spending

the winters on the Riviera, the summers fishing on the Scotch lochs. I had not been three months at Mentone before I began to improve both in general health and locally.

Bad air is not merely unhealthful but a mark of depravity, of decline from the golden age. Bowditch explodes on the subject; in earlier times, he says,

> The hearth-stone was really the gathering place for the family. Around that roaring "ventilating shaft," as it would be called now, the children conned their lessons or told their fairy tales, while their elders, perhaps, smoked their pipes; and yet, from the very nature of the arrangements, the air must have been purer than can by any means be found around our detestable airtight stoves, or those equally wretched apologies for comfort and health, the flues of the modern hot-air furnace, or coils for hot water and steam. Formerly there was less fear of drafts; no double windows were needed, but the father and his children drank in from their own hearth, warm, pure, but not over-heated air; while at the same time they were all fancy fed by the beautiful flame as it flickered and sang its quiet song all day. . . . Now all is altered.

It was a small step from the physical atmosphere to the social one. If darkness, poor ventilation, and crowding were consumption's handmaidens, the city was its mansion, fostering the conditions most favorable to it. The prevalence of tuberculosis became still another reason for despising urban blight, and that provoked a change in the way people viewed the disease itself. Once confined, at least in the popular imagination, to the refined and the educated, and thriving in isolation, it now became an urban disease, particularly a disease of the poor, whose attraction to the life of the streets thus earned hygienic as well as moral opprobrium:

> Cities exercise a mysterious attraction over the lower as well as the higher classes of mankind. It must be the feverish excitement of city life, the hope of greater social advancement—for the greater portion of the lower classes

in cities live as hard or harder lives than they would if similarly engaged in the country. No doubt the vitiated air breathed in cities, in the close crowded workshops, and in the closer and still more crowded sleeping rooms, gradually weakens constitutional powers, and constitutes one of the principle predisposing causes of Phthisis.

Though its crowds and bad air made the city a crucible of tuberculosis, it was also the place where the poor congregated, where oppressive economic conditions prevailed, where filth and ugliness constantly assaulted the senses. Health crusaders began to attack poor housing conditions, hence the landlords who permitted them to exist; poor working environments, hence the captains of industry who ran the factories; poor food and clothing, hence the unequal distribution of wealth in urban industrial America. Much of the early propaganda in the antituberculosis movement blames capitalism for the disease as directly as it does poor air and bad living conditions.

In 1913, for instance, the Cincinnati Anti-Tuberculosis League went so far as to produce a movie, *Darkest Cincinnati*, showing graphic vistas of misery, with unambiguous commentary about its causes:

Scene 5—A court between 4th and 5th Sts.
"A Sunday view of a court in this neighborhood. Filth and garbage from end to end. The stench is awful. Note the little girls carrying babies in their arms over piles of rotten garbage. Nearly all the property around this court belongs to one man."

Crowded tenements, windowless lodging rooms, dank airless courtyards, poor drainage were seen as increasing the landlord's income at the expense of human life. In a later scene, however, a child is seen sitting on her front step sobbing:

"And now we come to the other side of the picture where the hand of the good people through its agents is extended to distress caused by these conditions. Poor little Marie with a rose in her hand waiting for the nurse's call on mamma. How her face brightens when she sees the nurse from the Anti-Tuberculosis League."

The society reported large and enthusiastic crowds at every showing. Most of the movement's members came from the wealthier classes, and their benevolence could be as authoritarian as the economic imperialism of their factory-owning cousins and brothers-in-law. In 1912, responding to the problem of tuberculosis among the city's downtrodden, the New York Association for Improving the Condition of the Poor established a Home Hospital, in a section of the East River Homes on East Seventy-eighth Street. When someone eligible was stricken by tuberculosis, he and his whole family were admitted as a group, whereupon they underwent a long course of benevolent espionage and hygienic propaganda. If the family ate poorly, dressed inadequately, washed infrequently, slept with the windows shut or too many to a bed, these habits were quickly discovered and implacably stamped out by "instruction in precautions necessary to prevent the spread of tuberculosis within the family."

Implicit in the new impulse to attribute illness to the environment, however, was another new idea, which in reality amounted to an old one in new disguise. Where and how you lived were at least in part subject to your own control. If you chose to live in filth, or were too unambitious or too lazy to work yourself out of the crowded tenement districts, or preferred indolent dozing by the fireside to brisk walks in the fresh air and sunshine, you were bringing tuberculosis on yourself. And if, ultimately, you came down with it, you had only yourself to thank. Thus the disease could be taken once again as a constitutional weakness, though no longer as a desirable or admirable one. The consumptive's plight was no longer a sign of heavenly favor, but an earnest of genetic inferiority, an unwillingness or inborn inability to seek the conditions and perform the actions that might ward sickness off. Such a taint might be physical, moral, or psychological, but the distinction mattered little. If instinct tells you that pure air, good food, adequate clothing, cheerfulness, and temperance fight infection, what can be said of those who willfully bolt down hard-to-digest food, shut themselves up in overheated rooms, burden themselves with depressing thoughts, or, alternatively, gallivant about in flimsy ball gowns? "At the present time the extraordinary exposure of the person, when driving in party dresses to the ball in winter nights, is fearful, and the return home, after the whirl of the waltz, and when every fibre of the young frame is palpitating, is eminently hazardous."

Dying of the disease, whatever the cause of the infection, can in the end be taken as a proof of one's unfitness for life, the expression, inevitable conclusion, and just reward of inner weakness. The 1830s badge of delicate sensitivity had, in the increasingly practical, hard-minded, Darwinistic world of the 1870s, become a sign of corruption. Phthisis could be, and was, viewed as a benefit to mankind, pruning the unfit. "Viewed in this light, so far from Pulmonary Consumption being a dire inexplicable pestilence, striking indiscriminately the young and old, it becomes one of the provisions by which Providence has secured the integrity of the human race."

Still it was rare to push the idea to so extreme a conclusion; more commonly consumption emerges from a delicate nature, no longer as an efflorescence, but as self-destruction:

> We have seen cases where mental suffering, falling upon broad religious natures, has really ennobled the whole physical and mental life afterwards. Such natures do not usually succumb physically; they lose themselves in sympathy with others. Others, however, of less elevated characters are doubtless injured by suffering. Absorbed in themselves, becoming careless of their physical well-being, they allow themselves to neglect all these rules of health. . . . Consequently they may readily become victims of any disease to which . . . they may be in danger, and from which, without this superadded sorrow, they would have escaped. Among these diseases stands consumption.

The solution? The magazine publishing Bowditch's theories was, after all, the *Atlantic*; this was postabolitionist Boston. Little Eliza Herbert should come home from Italy, get out of bed, and do muscular good works:

> While requiring absolute attention to self-evident hygienic rules, we should endeavor to induce the sufferer to

seek relief from his or her own agony by becoming a ministering servant to the suffering of others. . . . Above all things prevent by every means in your power all brooding over past misfortune or sorrow. "Let the dead past bury its dead," and stimulate the unhappy invalid; and if this can be done, oftentimes consumption and all its kindred terrors will flee away.

Thus, whether an undiscovered microbe, exhalations in the atmosphere, or a fatal flaw in the constitution of the victim were at fault, it became increasingly unacceptable in the 1860s and 1870s simply to acquiesce in the fatality of consumption as inevitable. After all, the home could be ventilated, the slums cleared. Why couldn't the constitution of the sufferer be re-modeled as well? The 1870s saw the dawn of mind cure: the conviction that physical ills could yield to concentration and an optimistic outlook. The movement, in various forms, still sur-vives; some proponents, like Norman Vincent Peale, attribute only a sense of spiritual well-being and economic success to thinking healthily. But the pioneer of mind cure, Mrs. Mary Baker Glover (later Eddy), was not so vacillatingly modest.

Science and Health first appeared in 1875. It has been mer-cilessly satirized, most notably by Mark Twain, but what rend-ered it vulnerable to mockery was simply the clarity and forth-rightness with which it argued an idea that lurked behind much late-nineteenth-century thought, and behind the sanato-rium cure in particular. If, Mrs. Eddy proposed, the mind could intervene obscurely in the workings of the body, why not pursue the idea to its logical conclusion? There *is* no body. Only mind is real, and the material world, both in its pleasures and its ills, is illusory: "The era of science comes in on this statement and its proof, viz., that all is mind, and there is no matter. Sickness, sin, and death are creations of mortal mind, that Life, and Truth destroy."

Though many of them would no doubt have been scandal-ized to realize it, patients in the sanatoriums of the twenties and thirties, constantly exhorted to think positively, purge all melancholy thoughts, and sustain a happy frame of mind as a necessary part of the cure, were unconscious and sometimes unwilling spiritual heirs of Mrs. Eddy. "Why," an editorial in the *Mount McGregor Optimist* (a sanatorium magazine) rather cryptically asks, "cannot we all throw trouble off our shoulders by vigorously shaking the right and left shoulder, even tho it may appear that we are doing the enormous applesauce dance? At least we can have some fun during our stay on their roly poly ball, the planet earth." Betty MacDonald, admitted to a sanatorium near Seattle in the 1930s, found meals were always served with a card bearing a printed maxim; her first dinner came with the exhortation, "If you must be blue, be a bright blue."

Mind cure was an extension of, perhaps a reaction to, the widespread idea that sickness came from a weakness in one's constitution. If one's own being caused illness, might not that being somehow be trained to purge it? Mrs. Eddy's only real eccentricity was the firmness with which she made the claim that it could. Those same ideas lurked, in less blatant form, beneath the orthodox surface of many contemporary medical texts; they were to become dominant themes of the War on Consumption, the national publicity campaign that sought to turn that success into a national crusade.

In her way Mrs. Eddy was thus as much a scourge of sloppy thinking as Koch or Osler. But by their day, a bare ten years after Thoreau's exemplary death, ideas about the legendary disease that killed him were in flux. Old beliefs persisted, but new ones were in the air; painful research coexisted with wild guesses, mountebankery, and social philosophy. Consumption might be contagious; but then it might be hereditary. It might strike you through the very air you breathed, but it might lurk in your town, your neighborhood, your very family, not because these harbored pathogenic organisms, but because they *themselves* might cause sickness. Perhaps it struck from outside, and you were a blameless victim, but perhaps also it struck from within. If so, that might be a sign of preternatural sensitivity, or a proof that you were destined to end as genetic compost, unworthy to participate in the perpetuation of your species. Whatever your view of its cause, you might give in to your consumption, or you might battle it. If the latter, your choices were myriad: Piso's, Shiloh's, Radam's, Helmbold's, Schenck's patent remedies, sold at drugstores and advertised in the likes of the *New York Times,* as well as the penny press. All had a few mild herbs to stimulate the lungs and a few more potent narcotics to bludgeon the consciousness. Or you could undertake a hygienic regimen of life: fresh air, no fresh air, abundant food, skimpy food, absolute inactivity, a frenetic round of good works. You could play out your struggle with the captain of the men of death with your body as the principal battleground, or you could shift the action to your mind, convinced that aggressive optimism could heal the lungs and put death to a stand.

Your choices were bewilderingly many; theories about cause and cure were disorganized. The world was waiting for someone to forge a clear path through a forest of entangled images.

Then, in the spring of 1872, Edward Livingston Trudeau, a young doctor beginning his New York career, began to fall ill.

2

"The Greatest Battle Ever Fought":
Edward Livingston Trudeau and the War on Consumption

This crusade against the Great White Plague is the
greatest battle ever fought; the greatest game ever
played; the most deadly in earnest effort humanity ever
put forward to the benefit of humanity. Every one
engaged in the conflict should be alert, keen, alive.
                                    —ETHEL MCCORMICK
                            GRAND RAPIDS, MICHIGAN,
                                        WRITING IN THE
                        CONFIDENTIAL BULLETIN (1914)

Trudeau might have been the hero of a Henry James novel,
rich, well born in New York, raised and educated in Paris,
sophisticated, sensitive, accustomed to luxury, but primed for
tragedy. He had survived the death, in 1865, of a beloved
brother from tuberculosis; he had recently married and begun
to build a successful medical practice in New York.

Then he began to suffer from bouts of exhaustion. The
lymph glands on one side of his neck swelled and refused to
subside. During a summer residence on Long Island he
began experiencing intermittent attacks of illness that he attributed to malaria. Still, in the stoic, sickness-haunted 1870s,
that seemed small cause for alarm: "as nearly everybody had
malaria I . . . took quinine which, however, did little good."
Later, back in New York for the winter, he began running a
persistent fever, his temperature daily rising as high as 101
degrees.

At the insistence of his colleagues, he submitted to an examination. When it was concluded, the doctor said nothing. Trudeau ventured:

"Well, Dr. Janeway, you can find nothing the matter?" He looked grave and said, "Yes, the upper two-thirds of the left lung is involved in an active tuberculosis process."

I think I know something of the feelings of the man at the bar who is told he is to be hanged on a given date, for in those days pulmonary consumption was considered as absolutely fatal. I pulled myself together, put as good a face on the matter as I could, and escaped from the office after thanking the doctor for his examination. When I got outside . . . I felt stunned. It seemed to me the world had grown suddenly dark. The sun was shining, it is true, and the street was filled with the rush and noise of traffic, but to me the world had lost every vestige of brightness. I had consumption—that most fatal of diseases! Had I not seen it in all its horrors in my brother's case? It meant death and I had never thought of death before! Was I ready to die? How could I tell my wife, whom I had just left in unconscious happiness with the little baby in our new home? And my rose-colored dreams of achievement and professional success in New York! They were all shattered now, and in their place only exile and the inevitable end remained!

Following routine procedure, Dr. Edward Janeway no doubt heard in Trudeau's chest some or all of the telltale signs of advanced consumption: a dull sound when one tapped the chest above the clavicle; scarcely audible inhalation and prolonged exhalation; unsteady or "cogwheel" inspiration; the characteristic "râle," a clicking or gurgling rattle. Trudeau might be pardoned for making high drama of the scene in Janeway's office. Everyone who had tuberculosis and wrote about it did the same—to learn the truth was to be vouchsafed a revelation, an epiphany. Typhoid fever or smallpox announced themselves with a rapid, catastrophic onslaught of symptoms. But tuberculosis laid before you not a painful interlude but the whole remaining course of your earthly existence. Often in mockery of your wishes and ambitions, it rewrote your life; so the conventional response to it was not a series of entries on a medical chart but a resignation of the spirit, a lingering good-bye to all the preoccupations and diversions of earthly life.

Trudeau was fated to turn tuberculosis, however, from a malady into a career. More than any other individual, he transformed the imagery of consumption, drawing the American public after him. Jean Villemin and Robert Koch doubtless contributed more to the eventual conquest of the disease, but Trudeau's story, made famous by the movement he helped pioneer, created an atmosphere in which such a conquest seemed possible, even likely. He bridged the gap for the public between the old view of tuberculosis as a spiritual visitation, and the new, pragmatic spirit, determined to expose it for the purely physical syndrome it was and to conquer it.

After the dismaying news struck, Trudeau and his wife spent a hapless year trying to preserve what shreds of his health remained. A trip to South Carolina, which Janeway recommended, proved fruitless. They returned to New York in the spring of 1873, and in May, a week after his first son was born, he set off for what he thought would be a last hunting trip to the Adirondacks, which he had visited and fallen in love with two years before. His destination was Paul Smith's resort hotel, a few miles outside what is now Saranac Lake. At the time it was a relatively primitive place—drinking water, for instance, had to be hauled from a nearby spring in a pail—but it was beginning to be famous among New York's fashionable rich, who liked to listen to Smith's cagily rustic stories, eat his wife's home cooking, and hunt deer and bear in the woods behind his hostelry. Trudeau arrived there desperately ill, but hopeful: already, popular articles and books had begun to appear praising the area as pristine and healthful. At least as he remembered it in *An Autobiography,* the first sight of the mountains and the lake by Smith's encampment struck in him a sudden note of elation: "During the entire journey I had felt gloomy forebodings as to the hopelessness of my case, but, under the magic influence of the surroundings I had longed for, these all disappeared and I felt convinced I was going to recover."

He returned to New York much improved in September,

but a fall and winter there and in Minnesota produced a re-lapse, and the next summer, again desperate, he decided to move his whole family to the Adirondacks and remain through the winter. The story of their early years there, isolated and living in primitive conditions, has been told in his autobiography. Trudeau was befriended by Dr. Alfred Loomis, a New York physician and fellow hunting enthusiast whom he had met at Paul Smith's; Loomis, intrigued by the health-giving properties of the climate, had advised a tubercular patient to spend the winter there and was elated when both the patient and Trudeau stabilized and gradually improved. In 1879 he published a paper in the *Medical Record,* touting the Adiron-dacks as a health resort for the consumptive. Soon, the sick began to make their way to the mountains, via the few primi-tive modes of transportation then available, and as Trudeau's condition improved, he began to tend them. The village of Saranac Lake began to grow; invalids began to establish them-selves there and in outlying hamlets; and by 1883, the year after Koch's epoch-making discovery, Trudeau had decided to attempt to build a sanatorium. The first two-patient cottage, the Little Red, went up on a slope outside the village in 1884, effectively beginning the American War on Consumption.

It was to be a triumph of symbolism as much as the history of a real cure. The panic of Trudeau's diagnosis; his first hope-less decision to return to the Adirondacks; the miraculous (though in reality slow and painfully undramatic) improve-ment wrought by fresh air and rest; the opening, in 1885, of the Saranac Lake sanatorium, in hopes of bringing the same improvement to others—all this became the stuff of legend. Families read the story in fulsome public-service ads ("The Miracle of the Wilderness" was the title of a long-lived one), and it caught the popular imagination more viscerally than any other medical breakthrough in the early 1900s.

From the image of consumption that prevailed in the earlier nineteenth century, the change Trudeau brought about was a profound one. Before him, and from the time the disease first began to be scientifically described, the consumptive ap-

43

peared, even to medically trained observers, as removed from the common run of the human race, cut off from life as the rest of us live it, not so much corrupted as anointed by his disease. Somehow it conferred on him a premature flickering of the willowy transcendental afterlife early Victorian mortals were apparently hoping for. If on the one hand it meant sure death, on the other it also hastened the approach of what lay beyond. Trudeau had the good sense, even genius, to co-opt the very tradition he was replacing. In *An Autobiography,* before he himself is confronted with the diagnosis of consumption, he recounts at some length his brother's death from the same disease. The latter bears more than a passing resemblance to Paul Dombey and Little Eliza Herbert:

> From childhood he had been delicate, having a congenital heart trouble, and any over-exertion, excitement or fatigue caused his heart's action to become irregular and his nails and lips to turn blue. . . . [He] was a very strong, unselfish and beautiful character, deeply religious, and constantly trying to help me in the straight and narrow path from which I was apt to wander.

A consumptive of the old school, refined by disease, Trudeau establishes his own connection with that tradition by going on to emphasize his *own* delicacy and fragility when under the onslaught of the acute phases of his illness. But he was also about to pioneer a new, more robust ideology of consumption. The scene in Dr. Janeway's office was not to be the prelude to a similar tale of radiant decline; not the opening utterance in a long, languid farewell, but a turning point prefacing a triumph.

As consumptives, Trudeau presents both his brother and himself as frail and passive ("I have had ample opportunity in the past forty years to get used to illness and suffering; but it took me a long time to learn, imperfectly though it be, that acquiescence is the only way for the tuberculous invalid to conquer fate"). On the other hand, as doctor and survivor, Trudeau is robust, active, and aggressively masculine. Instead of languishing in Manhattan, he left for the mountains. As his health gradually improved, he became active again, gradually taking on more and more—new patients, the construction and operation of his sanatorium, the improvement of Saranac Lake's economic and spiritual life. Though schooled in an earlier, rather unmethodical medical tradition, he took pains to keep abreast of scientific advances, trained himself in laboratory techniques, and contributed to the advance of research in his field.

His patient's passivity became conquest, bed rest a military counterstrategy, a tactical retreat, the quiet first leg of the crusade. Ironically, by the time Trudeau adopted the rest cure, it had been long established in Europe and was actually on the decline there. But the great European sanatoriums had been, like the Hofrat Behrens's in *The Magic Mountain,* retreats for the middle and upper classes, luxury resorts. Trudeau's method was far more closely attuned to American obsessions: his hospital, first called the Adirondack Cottage Sanatorium, and renamed the Trudeau Sanatorium after his death, was a more rustic and democratic place, nearer to a summer (and winter) revival camp than a haunt of the rich. He charged patients only what they could afford to pay, served a range of sufferers, from Robert Louis Stevenson (who spent the fall and winter of 1887 and 1888 with him) to vagrants like a Brooklyn fruitseller, who somehow made their respective ways to Saranac and threw themselves on his mercy. To all equally he dispensed rest, pure air, good food, and a wholesome state of mind.

By the 1930s most sanatoriums printed magazines and distributed them to their patients. Like the typically titled *Optimist,* the house organ at the Metropolitan Life Insurance Company's corporate sanatorium at Mount McGregor, they were crammed with good cheer and uplift, touting the sanatorium not as a resting place for the enervated rich, but as a hearty popular alternative to the confinement of the industrial city. "Swing Into Action!" is the title of one article in the Spring 1938 issue of the *Optimist.* Another, by a patient, is equally affirmative: its sentiments would be as appropriate in a Dale

Carnegie course as in the rest cure. (In fact, the same issue of the *Optimist* records that the sanatorium library had just acquired *How to Win Friends and Influence People,* along with *Mathematics for the Million*, *Careers after Forty*, *Enjoyment of Laughter*, and *Finding Yourself in Your Work.*)

> Bring out your individual qualities. One never knows what he can accomplish until he tries. "Faint heart never won fair lady." Hop to it, you will be amazed at the hidden [power] lying dormant in that upper story, "Wake up and live" even tho you are temporarily on the side lines watching the world go by.
>
> Turn your present position in life to material advantage to yourself and to all with whom you come into contact. Bring forth into the open the best you have within you at all times. It will assist you to step over the rough spots, or apparent difficult bridges to cross. The entire situation is summed up in how you can respond or react to your own thoughts and desires. You can easily take one road to the depths of despair, or, just as easily another road to the height of contentment. Instructive, intelligent thinking should take up so much of your leisure time that you have not a moment to spare for that dread disease—*Nostalgia.*

In *An Autobiography,* the Adirondack wilderness acquires a dual symbolism. On the one hand it's Wordsworthian, soothing and succoring:

> On several occasions I have been taken to Paul Smith's from Saranac Lake in the spring so ill that my life was despaired of; and yet little by little, while lying out under the great trees, looking out on the lake all day, my fever has stopped and my strength slowly begun to return. Last spring—1914—at Saranac Lake I was so ill and weak that I had ceased, for the first time in my life, even to care to live any longer. I arrived at Paul Smith's at the end of June on a mattress, which had been placed in the automobile of a good friend, and the same feeling of hope and courage came back when I was carried up to my airy porch in the little cottage, with the stillness of the great forest all about me, the lake shimmering in the sunlight.

But it was also a place to be conquered, of challenges to be overcome. Trudeau's first inkling of improvement came, by his own admission, *not* during bed rest but on the lake, during a hunting trip; the body turns a corner when its owner wins, however vicariously, a battle:

> As I lay comfortably on the soft boughs in the stern of the boat, with my rifle in reach across the gunwale, my spirits were high and I forgot all the misery and sickness I had gone through in the past two months. Then, on a point about two hundred yards away I saw two deer: a buck and a doe were feeding. I never sat up, but rested my rifle on the side of the boat and fired at the buck who, after a few jumps, fell dead at the edge of the woods. . . . I got back quite triumphant to the hotel.

Despite the fact that Trudeau was among the first prominent American physicians to accept Koch's discovery and played a vital role in disseminating it both to the medical community and the general public, his regimen for the cure strikes primitive chords, harmonizes science with something more atavistic. Patent medicines were, finally, driven from the marketplace by the emerging medical establishment in the early 1900s. But purging the materia medica of Buchu Extract and weed killer doubling as a germicide depended on a successful appeal to the American public. Science had to grab the popular imagination as firmly as the bottled remedies espoused by Piso, Schenck, and Radam had. The tubercle bacillus had to be repackaged for the public taste before practical knowledge of it could seize the collective mind; medical complexities had to be made part of a familiar and accessible context.

Trudeau achieved this; he was a pioneer of socially responsible hucksterism. He caught the nation's attention by deserting the city, forging his way into the wilderness, meeting its challenges and emerging a stronger man; repeating in a medical context the story of the whole American experience, endorsing in the process its suspicion of the cities and its love of open space.

But the popular imagination, reliably conservative, was not ready to sacrifice the romantic view of the tubercular invalid as etherealized wraith. Somehow this newer view of consumption as an urban disease, a product of crowding, filth, poverty, and overwork, had not to replace but to meld with the picturesque ills of Paul Dombey, Francine, and Little Eliza Herbert. Thus the genius behind the Little Red, the one-room bungalow that, in 1885, began the history of Trudeau's Adirondack Cottage Sanatorium. A few other American tuberculosis hospitals preceded it, and hundreds of others were to imitate it beginning in the 1890s. There would be variations from hospital to hospital, but the routine Trudeau established at Saranac Lake became the model for all.

As he constituted it, the cure was not a hospital stay but a way of life, not a giving in to the onslaught of illness but a conversion to a nearly religious regimen of health. The name of the National Tuberculosis Association's popular magazine, the *Journal of the Outdoor Life,* conveys the idea that the sanatorium was not just a hospital but a community, a microcosm among the sick of the world of the well.

While Trudeau drew many of his ideas from the *English Practitioner,* which in turn followed Gustav Herrmann Brehmer's pioneer sanatorium in Silesia, he chose the Adirondacks for reasons having little to do with any existing theory of the disease. His motivations were more visionary than scientific, and as he describes them they sound more like the dreams of a utopian idealist than a medical pragmatist; they are practical only in the sense that they apparently worked.

> Many a beautiful afternoon, for the first four winters after I came to Saranac Lake, I had sat for hours alone while hunting, facing the ever-changing phases of light and shade on the imposing mountain panorama at my feet, and dreamed the dreams of youth; dreamed of life and death and God, and yearned for a closer contact with the Great Spirit who planned it all, and for light on the hidden meaning of our troublous existence. . . . This spot always has had a wonderful influence on me, and it is not to be

wondered at that I decided almost at once to place the first little wooden building of my proposed Sanitarium on it.

Strange words for a clinician. But in fact as the hospital grew, it became less and less like a medical facility, more and more like a town: a cluster of buildings in many sizes and styles, arrayed on a planned landscape, a self-sufficient economic unit. Thirty years later, as Trudeau describes it, it might have been mistaken for a small city; and in this it was like any major rural sanatorium between 1910 and 1940.

The mountains now look down on a different scene. The old boulders and the rough pasture have disappeared, and macadamized roads, sloping grass lawns, flower beds and ornamental shrubs have taken their place. The Sanitarium has grown to be a picturesque little village. It comprises thirty-six buildings scattered over the entire hillside between the north and south gates, a distance of about three quarters of a mile. The patients' cottages are grouped about the large Administration Building, and other cottages for the heads of departments are clustered together at the south entrance, near which are the stables, barns, and the big fire-proof laundry. In addition to the patients' cottages, there are many other buildings which represent various activities: a nurses' home for the Training School, an infirmary for bed-ridden patients, a post office, a colonial brick and marble library building, a reception and medical building with offices, laboratory and x-ray department, a recreation pavilion for amusements and entertainments, a workshop building where the patients are taught fancy leather-work, book-binding, brass work and framemaking as a recreation and as graded exercise, and a beautiful stone chapel.

The complexity of the facility is striking: housing divides along class lines; there are places for work, learning, recreation, and worship; there is even a hospital within the hospital town, in the pavilion for bedridden patients.

Where once the hospital had been a place of horror, a repository for the hopeless—destitute, dark, filthy, hidden as far as possible from the sites of normal human activity, the sanatorium transformed it into an extension of everyday life, a place where living, albeit tubercular living, went on much as it did everywhere. If to the cynical observer its completeness in isolation and its self-sufficiency might suggest a leper colony, for the patient it proved that he was not cut off from the world, only leading a parallel life in special circumstances. Turning out wampum belts and crocheted hot-water bottle covers may not have been rewarding work in itself, but for the convalescent it provided a link with his past and, he hoped, future, productive life.

By the late 1880s Trudeau's little city of health was flourishing. Patients were beginning to flock to it, and it could point to successful outcomes, though the cure at this stage in its history was not as systematic as it was later to become; it was not the product of a clearly thought-out rationale. Trudeau had come from the city to the mountains and had, thanks to bracing air, uplifting scenery, and a simple life, got better. His grandson, Dr. Francis Trudeau, compares his state of mind at the time to that of an athlete, who, without a detailed knowledge of anatomy or physiology, simply listens to the signals his body gives him as he competes, and behaves accordingly. Early patients at the Adirondack Cottage Sanatorium followed no ironclad regimen. Sometimes they rested, sometimes they exercised; Trudeau experimented with novel therapies as they became available, though no single method ever dominated.

If matters had rested here, Trudeau might never have been heard from again, and lived out his life among a few patients in happy isolation, surrounded by the protecting mountains. But he had come from New York, retained his contacts with it, and publicized his success among its civic leaders. His old friend and physician, Dr. Alfred Loomis, continued to send patients to him from New York; his article about the Adirondacks in the *Medical Record* had publicized the area as a health resort, kindling awareness of it among physicians along the Eastern Seaboard; in the 1890s this awareness began to extend to the public at large, as articles appeared in the popular press. And the sanatorium, as it grew, began to demand larger and larger infusions of money, since it was never supported fully by its patients, whose means were mostly modest.

Consequently Trudeau began making annual trips to New York, importuning his rich and influential connections for contributions. Trudeau's evident charm turned the trick, and donations flowed; but, perhaps more important, his success in the mountains, spoken of glowingly in the city, helped establish tuberculosis as a fashionable charity: the lure of the wilderness, combined with the prospect of an effective war on mankind's leading killer, intrigued and attracted urban philanthropists. Donations flowed in, and cadres of people interested in the campaign against consumption and the sanatorium experiment began to appear in major Eastern cities.

By 1890 these groups had come to include both physicians and interested laymen, and the antituberculosis movement began to grope toward a formal organization. In New York, Dr. Hermann M. Biggs began goading the city government into a planned campaign against the disease; in Philadelphia in 1892, Dr. Lawrence Flick organized the first voluntary association, the Pennsylvania Society for the Prevention of Tuberculosis. There were, of course, forces behind this rising enthusiasm other than Trudeau's fledgling success at Saranac Lake—scientific advances, though not yet at the point of offering a reliable cure, had suggested that the old enemy could be conquered, especially since the mode of transmission had come to be understood. But Trudeau gave such theoretical hopes a firm foundation in myths that appealed viscerally not only to the professional medical man but to the responsible community leader. The sick, it now appeared, could be sent beneficially to a health-giving retreat in the wilderness. The well, remaining in the cities, could be exhorted to give up behavior that, it was now certain, fostered the spread of contagion. And both enterprises required the cooperation of professionals and amateurs in the kind of voluntary movement the French commentator Alexis de Tocqueville had long before remarked as a uniquely

American phenomenon. The prospect was not the less inviting because, in defining its spirit, Trudeau had invoked values sure to appeal to the American ruling class—optimism, pragmatism, self-reliance—and had further confirmed the usefulness of a uniquely American landscape.

Spurred by a now-enthusiastic national press, voluntary antituberculosis associations began springing up across the country: by 1901 there were eight statewide associations and eleven local societies, and it had become clear that the movement needed a national voice. There were various false starts and disputes, many revolving around the provocative question of whether the national organization would be controlled by doctors or laymen, but finally, on June 6, 1904, the National Association for the Study and Prevention of Tuberculosis met for the first time, in Atlantic City; Trudeau, unsurprisingly and justly, was elected as the first president. After a prolonged ovation, he spoke to the group:

> I cannot find words suitable to express my appreciation for the great honor you have done me. . . . While struggling for so many years alone and in a remote region with the tuberculosis problem about me, my wildest fancy never pictured the possibility of such a wide-spread and earnest movement as this.

Once it consolidated, the association embarked on a national campaign of propaganda and education that was to blanket the country for the next fifty years. Though it supported research, and to a limited extent involved itself in relief for the sick, it resolved after some initial debate to concentrate on the prevention of tuberculosis, leaving treatment to the sanatoriums.

In its early years, between 1908 and 1913, the association issued a mimeographed newsletter to its members, the *Confidential Bulletin,* which became a wellspring of the imagery the movement was to enforce upon the public in the ensuing decades. It soon became clear that in concentrating on prevention, the association had perforce launched itself on a course of publicity and image making. The War on Consumption was in fact a national mobilization of opinion through advertising. Unlike the Schencks and the Radams, the leaders of the movement were eminently high-minded, respectable representatives of Progressivism. But whereas the patent-medicine men had been content with a limited share of the market, the national association and its local affiliates needed, by definition, to monopolize it. The schemes outlined in the early numbers of the *Confidential Bulletin* are designed not only to publicize the War on Consumption but also to assure that the view of tuberculosis (and for that matter of good health) it espoused was uniform from city to city, state to state. National conceptions about consumption had to be coordinated; tuberculosis thus took on a further dimension as one of the earliest unifiers of the national consciousness, an early instance of homogenized image making on a countrywide scale.

This demanded an exercise of power more diffuse than, but just as manipulative as, that practiced on sanatorium inpatients. The local association in Saint Louis formulated a uniform neighborhood-by-neighborhood campaign, built around a simple lecture. And, as one issue of the bulletin indicates, the drumming up of attendance was accomplished with formidable and apparently effective hoopla:

> Dodgers are distributed from house to house and cards placed in all the store windows. . . . Conspicuous on each card is the slogan, "Listen for the bombs." Then commences the aerial cannonade and at five-minute intervals the bombs are exploded. They are thrown high in the air and the report can be heard for blocks. People speedily come when they hear them. . . . The dodgers do not specify that the meeting is for the purpose of a lecture on tuberculosis, but . . . their curiosity is aroused and they come in droves. . . .

The *Bulletin* was confidential not because it hid any grave secrets or explosive gossip but simply out of solidarity among the few banding together to aid, and incidentally to control, the many. Its ideal is health but its constant theme is power.

Early issues exhort health activists to enlist industrialists in their campaigns, because of the influence they exert over their workers.

> Find a busy man whose heart prompts him and whose standing in the community will enable him to call a meeting of the heads of the largest manufactories, department stores, hotels, laundries and other institutions. . . . Present the plan to these men and draw out discussion—they are brainy men and every one will contribute valuable ideas.

Drumming up publicity "along lines somewhat similar to those followed by a big traveling circus," the New York State Health Department canvassed not only industrialists and doctors but the clergy, who exhorted their parishioners from the pulpit. Bold posters went up on streetcars; there were billboards, handbills, and prominently displayed maps on which "black pins indicate the approximate location of deaths in five, ten or fifteen year periods."

Local campaigns focused primarily on one thing: a home version of Trudeau's Outdoor Life—pure air, good food, clean morals, and a cheerful frame of mind. Though not enforced, as in the sanatorium, by doctors and nurses, the rules were peremptory. As part of its fresh-air drive, for example, the Minnesota association mounted "a determined crusade against nailed-on storm windows. . . . The head of every household where storm windows are found fastened on in such a way as not to be readily opened, will be requested by the local committee to make the necessary changes." Whether the committee members merely inquired politely or prowled the shrubbery in search of nailed-on windows is not clear, but its officiousness is. The Texas Anti-Tuberculosis Society published the following bossy public-service announcement in the *Dallas News*:

> DON'T SPIT on the floor of your shop.
> WHEN YOU SPIT, spit in the gutters or in a spittoon.
> Have your own spittoons half full of water, and clean them out at least once a day with hot water.

DON'T COUGH without holding a handkerchief or your hand over your mouth.

DON'T live in rooms where there is no fresh air.

DON'T work in rooms where there is no fresh air.

DON'T sleep in rooms where there is no fresh air.

Keep at least one window open in your bedroom day and night.

Fresh air helps to kill the consumption germ.

Fresh air helps to keep you strong and healthy.

DON'T eat with soiled hands—wash them first.

DON'T DRINK WHISKEY, beer, or other intoxicating drinks; they will do you no good, but will make it harder for you to get well.

DON'T SLEEP IN THE SAME BED with anyone else, and, if possible, not in the same room.

Some of these dicta are germane to the prevention of tuberculosis but others seem more moral than hygienic, aimed at reforming the workingman's behavior even as they shored up his health. Indeed, the antituberculosis movement concerned itself with all forms of social improvement; health and personal conduct intertwined. Along with its stock lectures on tuberculosis, housing, and working conditions, the American Institute of Social Service offered another on "THE AMUSEMENT PROBLEM . . . Snares of Amusements. Saloons. Dance Halls. Burlesque Theaters." If the early, pre-Trudeauvian consumptive was implicitly an aristocrat, the new, city-dwelling, poor patient, inferior in other ways, must fall short in morals as well; and his doctor should be vigilant. Moreover, at a time when labor was becoming increasingly restive, the unquestionably benevolent hygiene movement was preaching that the worker's best interest lay in the direction of passive obedience. Small wonder that factory owners were easily persuaded to join the antituberculosis movement. Might not the laborer, trained to obey the hygiene worker, become more amenable to orders from the foreman?

Predictably, power also became an issue between the movement and others competing for its audience. It had borrowed many of its methods from business; business, ever enterprising, struck back. In 1910 a company called the White Cross League appeared, selling soap, toilet articles, and flavoring extracts. The owners claimed all their profits would be donated to tuberculosis relief, but the national association reported that only twelve cents of every dollar earned went to consumptives. In 1912 the McKinley Memorial Hospital League solicited donations for a projected tuberculosis hospital and outlined a plan for issuing stamps like the national association's recently instituted Red Cross (later Christmas) seals. After an investigation the association dyspeptically announced that the McKinley League was run by "individuals for the most part of questionable responsibility." The woman in charge of their field work, "a Miss Mary Rossiter, had been arrested and convicted of larceny and served a term in the penitentiary some years ago."

Such chicanery was disturbing, of course, but a sign of the crusade's success—nothing negligible would have drawn so many predators, and none of them stemmed the tide. Stock lectures multiplied. In 1913 the association, formally assuming—in fact implicitly outdoing—the original crusades, adopted as its insignia not a single but a double red cross, the logo still used by its successor, the American Lung Association. Characteristically, the association was concerned that the symbol be absolutely uniform wherever it was used. All arms of the cross were to be pointed; the two cross arms were to be equal in length; the lower leg seven units, the arms three units on either side and one and one-half units apart; and the staff above the arms two and one-half units high. The American Civic Association chartered Fly-Fighting Committees in Washington, D.C., Grand Rapids, and other cities. Fly-catching contests were initiated among schoolchildren, the collector of the most flies, living or dead, being awarded ten dollars. (A boy in Grand Rapids caught twenty-six quarts.) In the last issue of the *Confidential Bulletin*—it was to survive under another name but lose its confidential status as the association recruited more and more participants—Ethel McCormick, also of Grand Rapids, wrote a ringing call to arms:

This crusade against the Great White Plague is the greatest battle ever fought; the greatest game ever played; the
most deadly in earnest effort humanity ever put forward
to the benefit of humanity. Every one engaged in the
conflict should be alert, keen, alive.

By the 1920s the movement had grown into an industry.
Sanatoriums proliferated; health campaigns burgeoned. The
Metropolitan Life Insurance Company lent both its prestige
and its formidable economic power to the campaign, building
its own company sanatorium at Mount McGregor in Saratoga
County, New York, on the site where Ulysses S. Grant had died.

The dedication ceremonies, in June 1914, were notable even
for a movement given to trumpet blasts and clarion calls, in the
fervor with which they wedded the causes of hygiene, social
welfare, commercial self-confidence, and evangelical religion.
John R. Hegeman, the president of Metropolitan Life, wrote
from a summer retreat at Marienbad:

> Neither prosperity, nor its consequent power to
> achieve would, in any degree, have availed without the
> *Disposition,* wed to the *Determination,* of Officers and
> Directors alike, to rise to the full height of opportunity
> and possibility.
> All have been animated by PAUL's admonition—"We
> that are *strong* ought to bear the infirmities of the
> weak." . . .
> Thus, without strain of language, may Mount McGre-
> gor, already hallowed by historic association, be deemed
> as consecrated ground. May the light of inspiration and
> influence that shall beam from its sunlit crest be a verita-
> ble *"light that never fails."*

The citation of Paul here is apropos; he was the evangelist most
appropriate to the crusade, in his emphasis on conversion, his
militancy, and his division of the world into opposing forces of
dark and light.

And, in fact, the fervor of Hegeman's dedication, if grandiloquent, was real. The company was for the next several decades to devote a major portion of its resources to the eradication of tuberculosis. Apart from Mount McGregor, it conducted a large-scale national advertising campaign of its own, publishing numerous handouts. The formidable forces of kitsch were unleashed on the public. A 1915 pamphlet, *A War on Consumption,* includes in its rather overfreighted cover illustration all the strands that had been woven, since the 1870s, into popular understandings of the disease.

In the background a smoke-shrouded landscape glowers; in the foreground a sunlit meadow, shaded by flowering trees. (Most of the flowers form a background to the title, A WAR ON CONSUMPTION, as if to soften its dire import.) The contrast is multivalent. The background is the grim past, the imprisonment of the city, disease, industrial slavery, hopeless financial insecurity; the foreground is the glorious future, the pure air of the country, health, freedom from grinding toil, the security of a policy issued by Metropolitan Life.

A procession of faceless sufferers, who, as they emerge from the shadows, become beaming survivors, is led away by a female figure robed in white. Hygeia? Her gown bears the double-barred cross of the National Tuberculosis Association, but more prominent is a white banner she holds aloft, bearing the symbol of the Metropolitan Life Insurance Company—the clocktower on the corporate headquarters in New York, crowned by its famous beacon.

We are being reminded that although fresh air and sunlight may help, and the nationwide campaign may serve a worthy end, the shining light in the crusade is corporate—not the old-fashioned smokestack business with its oppressed workers and airless factories, but the benevolent corporation, in the Pauline tradition so eloquently affirmed by President Hegeman. Disease and death, hitherto the territory of the professions, the clergy, and the victim himself, are henceforth being colonized by business. Consumption (meaning an economic activity) was coming into use just as its medical meaning was beginning to fade, giving way to the more technical "tuberculosis." The disease was giving way, becoming more than a problem for a science and a terror to its victims; it was becoming the basis of an economy.

And an ordered economy at that. A glimpse at the beaming throngs who follow Hygeia into the light proves it. The crowd is biblical in its universality—the old, the young, the hale, the classically infirm. A bespectacled blind man, a dapper business-man, sober matron, young mother, hooded spinster, babe in arms. And it behaves itself; it follows; it recognizes hierarchy, and makes sure the proper distinctions are preserved. The males all appear to wear roughly contemporary clothes, but the females wear rather antiquated (appropriately backward?) nineteenth-century costume. The families tread firmly in the main path; the apparent spinsters are wandering on the peripheral verdure.

The picture is divided in the center by a river, so that foreground and background are clearly marked off as above and below. The grateful hordes pass over a bridge, establishing a clear border between past and future, sickness and health, ignorance and enlightenment, superstition and science, festering city and fragrant countryside, fatalistic despair and cheerful optimism. Also, the river flows between the double-barred cross and the Light That Never Fails: business and voluntarism cooperate, but remain apart, business retaining a superior place. Perhaps the artist was unconscious of what teemed beneath the surface of his design. No matter: if a mind is deeply enough impregnated with a complex of values, every shape it dreams up will emerge saturated with them.

The very center of the picture, however, is neither Hygeia nor the corporate logo, but two gamboling children, and that highlights another fixation of the War on Consumption. Tuberculosis was sometimes pictured, though inaccurately, as a disease of youth; but the movement's interest in children rather reflected its preoccupation with educating the public, hence of adopting the methods of the schoolroom, and, perhaps, consequently infantilizing its audience. Children listen, trust, and can be led—in that respect they serve as an example to adults.

And, at the same time, they can be relied upon to arouse the adult's otherwise perhaps passive emotions and engage them on behalf of the campaign. Thus antituberculosis propaganda is at its most quintessential in the nursery.

Childhood plays the same role in the early history of the imagery of tuberculosis that it does in the illustration: not dominant but ubiquitous. The great tubercular victims in the Victorian and early modern novel—Beth March, Little Nell, Paul Dombey—are often children, or—Mimi, Milly Theale—overgrown children, crypto-children. In his autobiography Trudeau dwells at length on his own childhood and that of his nameless, doomed, beloved brother, implying the illness was somehow sown in youth. In his 1869 *Atlantic* article Bowditch surveyed consumptives of all ages, but his imagination was also most captured by children:

> We must confess the sad and unwelcome truth that [some children] are doomed to an early death. By the diseased condition of the parents, sometimes, alas! due to their own or their ancestors' previous excesses, the tender bodies of the children are so tainted that life becomes a burden. We have often seen in such cases the terrible vindication of the power of the old Mosaic law, "For the sins of the fathers are visited upon the children unto the third and fourth generation." Such children die early; and this is exactly right. The race would constantly deteriorate were it otherwise. For there is no greater proof of Divine foresight than the law which certainly prevails, that only to strength and perfect health belongs the highest life, which alone has as its birthright the will and the power to contribute to the continuance of the human race.

The mixture of ideas here is remarkable. Darwin and God collaborate in severing the reproductive lines of the weak by destroying the innocent, who, expiring, enact a morally improving spectacle for the sensitive observer.

The child is a symbolic vessel for the whole human race, its possibilities and its vulnerabilities. In his dependence on others, the child is already a convenient image for the consumptive, passive and doomed without the help of his guardians. He is innocent, but, through original sin, he bears the stain of guilt. His potential is greater than the adult's, but so is his frailty. He makes, when one is needed, a convenient scapegoat, connected intimately with the community whose sin he is to be made to bear, yet separated from it by his immaturity.

No wonder if a symbolically fraught disease should intersect with a symbolically fraught stage of life, producing a disproportionate share of tuberculosis literature either about or aimed at children. They were, after all, a captive audience as adults weren't. They *liked* to follow. They could be convinced of their vulnerability and inoculated with the spirit of the crusade, their naïve enthusiasm made militant. But how could naïve imaginations be transformed into accurate knowledge and a mastery of practical measures against the disease?

The *Journal of the Outdoor Life,* the popular magazine for consumptives and their loved ones, responded to this concern by aiming some of its articles at children. These are useful to us here because they reveal the underlying themes of the movement in bold relief; like good fairy tales, they make the latent scarifying manifest. The November 1915 issue included "Two Morality Interludes for Children," by Professor George M. P. Baird of the University of Pittsburgh. They were intended for performance in schools during Tuberculosis Week, and particularly on Children's Health Crusade Day.

That there are two of them is already symbolic of the movement, its penchant for dualism, its habit of making contrasts—light and dark, city and country, past and future. The first playlet, "The Theft of Thistledown," subtitled "A Faery Interlude," aims at handling its subject lightly, and is pitched at younger children. The second, "The Narrow Door," is, as its title implies, a gloomier piece, directed presumably at the moroser sensibilities of adolescents.

"The Theft of Thistledown" puts the young child's love of fairy lore to the service of health education. Queen Maeve holds a fairy court. Attendant pixies cavort before her and recount their exploits.

> I've been with the painters of rainbows,
> Who ply their bright trade in the skies
> With fleecy white cloudlets for brushes
> And the souls of the flowers for dyes.

But one of the pixies, Thistledown, has visited earth, a forbidden place. He speaks, significantly, in prose: "I only intended to sail above it in my gossamer ship, but the earth air was so heavy with the poison smoke of cities that it made me horribly thirsty." Landed, Thistledown seeks nectar-bearing flowers but finds only artificial ones, manufactured by a wretched family, "a weary earth mother and six hungry looking children." Overcome by toil, the mother neglects her baby:

> All alone in a grimy basket, wrapped and smothered in dirty rags, lay this earth-baby, blinking its rheumy red eyes at the blazing summer sun and sucking, between its sobs, at a bottle full of that nasty drink, which men call tea.

Not that the mother inflicts such horrors on her child intentionally; it's a matter of conditions beyond her control:

> When the baby cried or screamed louder than usual she would look at it over her bowed shoulder with a hopeless wistful glance; say, "hushaby, hushaby, hush," two or three times, and then go on making muslin daisies. Once she took a sticky bit of candy from the mouth of one of the children and gave it to the baby. That kept it quiet for awhile, but the flies soon gathered on its smudgy, little, pimpled red face and it began to whine again.

Baird no doubt meant this sudden realism to shock his young audience out of its presumed enchantment and into recognition of the squalor around them. Echoing that plunge from fairyland to earth, Thistledown, having sympathetically rescued the infant and fetched it up before Queen Maeve, is condemned by her to take its place on earth until

> The world growing better, mankind
> Shall give to its children one half
> Of the care that's now lavished on gold.

The story's abruptly nasty turn from Arthur Rackham to Upton Sinclair has a purpose, to show the contrast between Thistledown, Maeve, Burr, Bramble, and Blueberry and the world the audience really lives in, beset by disease, filth, and poverty. The dualism is crude, but it also has a latent dimension: it illustrates something about human ambiguousness toward disease. On the one hand we must detach ourselves from the invalid, persuade ourselves that the world he lives in isn't ours: we are the charmed elves, he the grubbing sufferer; we get the verse while he gets the pustules. Yet the sick can't be excluded—to do so would be inhuman, and would also belie the universal human awareness that anyone may suddenly become ill and die. Just as theories about consumption did, the playlet moves symbolically from poetry to realism, from Arcadia to the city slums; it brings idealism to earth. The closing appeal, "And you, O people of the earth, if there be any among you who can help in this great work of saving earth-babies, I pray you join with us; for it is a mighty task and will require the hearts and brains and purses of us all for its swift doing," draws a practical moral, but the forces at work underneath the story are more exotic. The children must identify both with the privileged and the downtrodden, must see themselves both as potential victims and potential rescuers.

As was not the case with most other major diseases, tuberculosis could present intermittent and ambiguous symptoms: a successful outcome demanded that the patient make an act of faith both in the existence of his disease and in the efficacy of the rest cure. So in a sense both the warriors against tuberculosis and its beneficiaries had to be recruited; doctor and patient had to be at once identified with and distinguished from each other. Albeit unconsciously, "The Theft of Thistledown" prepares its audience for that paradox.

"The Narrow Door" is altogether grimmer; in it Baird gives free rein to a taste for morbid lyricism. As Grieg plays in the background, two sisters, Vita and Hygeia, spin. They are gloomy, and with reason, because behind them "yon dark shape, our brother Mors" is claiming more and more young lives.

> O, sister life, when we began to spin
> In the great golden morning of the world,
> The fibres were lithe wires and broke not
> In spinning, but served long their destined end
> In the clock of God, or His bow-string, or
>   i' the lute
> Wherewith he makes eternal melody.

But now, Hygeia says, "ignorance of the wise, gold-lust, neglect," and "the love unschooled to guard its own" have sent more and more to Mors and through the Narrow Door. Moreover, "the hollowed threshold of the narrow door/ Is worn by little feet."

In this piece the audience can't identify with the immortals: Hygeia and Vita are too abstract to permit that. When they finish their prologue, some listless children march onto the stage: a Child Leader, Paolo, Laura, Maria, Paulus, and Elain. They don't speak but carry "crystal spheres which they wave, offering-wise, to the rhythm of soft music."

One by one the children show signs of fatigue. An offstage Voice calls Paulus, who "arises painfully and slowly goes out through the narrow door." Then Maria. Then Laura. Then Paolo. Then Elain.

> O women who spin, have you seen
> Our playfellows, Paulus the tall,
> Golden-haired Laura, Paolo,
> And gentle Maria? They danced
> But a moment ago by our side
> And now they are gone.

In a mournful conclusion Hygeia and Vita deliver to the few survivors a brief lecture. Death, they explain, is not the enemy:

> Mankind, not Death, is the stern foe of children!
> It wins its gold through the toil of little fingers;
> Poisons the sweet blue air; lets fever burn
> From court to crowded court; taints meat and drink.

The children in the audience are at once being threatened with death and recruited into the army of social betterment. The content of the sober vision is the same as that of the frivolous one in the companion piece: consumption is a place where opposites meet. You are Paulus, Paolo, and Elain; but if you put aside your crystal sphere and join the crusade, you may avert death yourself and save others as well. The Child Leader marches up to the apron and exhorts the audience.

> O men and children of men,
> It lies in your power to rear
> A barrier, builded of love,
> Across the dim doorway; and stop
> The criminal waste of young life.

The child crosses a border. In the act of confronting consumption, he confronts the interdependence of life and death, and comes of age. Thistledown joins the human race and faces his own mortality; the Child Leader joins the National Tuberculosis Association and battles it.

Traditionally tuberculosis was thought a disease particularly apt to strike just at the moment one entered maturity. The shadow falls across a path just begun, like Trudeau's or Hans Castorp's in *The Magic Mountain,* and diverts the voyager elsewhere; it blurs the border between childhood and adulthood, dependence and responsibility. Baird's two playlets are about exactly those obscured borders; are attempts to clear them. That they're silly is beside the point—they are silly about, and hence call up, a profound theme.

Between 1872 and 1915 the health crusaders didn't succeed in eradicating consumption. But they did succeed in turning it from an angelic visitation or an amorphous terror into a system of clear and easily understood though contradictory symbols. These in turn reflected themes and contradictions in American life: to have tuberculosis was to be American only more so, to dramatize in your own body the traumas of the nation at large, to internalize contemporary history. Hence the preoccupation with belles lettres, the strenuously literary language affected by everyone in the movement, from Trudeau and Bowditch to Baird. It was natural and inevitable if you conceive that their main aim was not discovery of scientific facts but the construction of an image. Their gift, and more particularly Trudeau's, was a tough but endurable way to cope with a disease, to understand it as a reflection of the world around it, without totally ignoring the biological discoveries that were rendering it more and more susceptible to the scrutiny of science.

Tuberculosis was, of course, everywhere, but only America made it a national obsession, exaggerating its terrors, then exaggerating the degree to which those terrors could be conquered. Though it deals only glancingly with consumption, the first edition of Mary Baker Eddy's *Science and Health* echoes this. On the one hand it is crammed with announcements that Mind can conquer illness: "sickness, sin and death are creations of mortal mind, that Life, and Truth destroy"; on the other, it is a cornucopia of woeful afflictions—ladies who breathe poorly when the wind is east, leaky livers, digestions able to tolerate only one three-inch-square slice of bread per day. In his determination to think positively while beset by inward and outward terrors, the late-nineteenth-century consumptive, following the trail blazed by Trudeau, was making manifest the latent life of his country, claiming optimism but seized with terror at signs of necrosis and impending apocalypse. When he left the scene of his diagnosis in New York, Boston, or Chicago and headed for a sanatorium, whether in the Adirondacks or a suburb of his own city, the experience he was embarking on was a microcosm of America in the early twentieth century.

3

"Rules and a Daily Routine":
The Rise of the Sanatorium

The process of the "cure" in tuberculosis, as well as in many other diseases, depends largely on your own body tissues, and the nursing and medical care which you receive are designed to strengthen your body's fight against the disease.

Hence the need for rules and a daily routine. The rules and the routine by which you will live here are designed to help you, as a patient, to get well as promptly as possible, and to indicate how you . . . can contribute to the common good of the group living at the Sanatorium and make our life together friendly, considerate, and free from needless worry.

—*Instructions and Information for Patients,*
METROPOLITAN LIFE INSURANCE
COMPANY SANATORIUM,
MOUNT MCGREGOR, N.Y. (1942)

The first modern tuberculosis sanatorium was a monument to a wrongheaded theory. In the 1840s Gustav Herrmann Brehmer, a Silesian physician, observed that consumption rarely occurred at altitudes above 1,600 feet. He reasoned that living in the thinner air of the mountains made the heart work harder and strengthened it, concluding that tuberculosis struck when the heart, weak and sluggish, failed to pump away poisonous accumulations from the lungs. If, he thought, the tubercular were brought to an invigorating mountain landscape, encouraged to embark on a carefully supervised program of graded exercise, fed herculean Teutonic meals (five of them a day), and plunged regularly under cold showers (Brehmer's sister was a hydrotherapist), they would thrive and recover, their revitalized hearts purifying their debilitated lungs.

At first his plan made but slow headway. By the mid-nineteenth century the Prussian medical bureaucracy was already well organized and insisted on clearing all health-care projects; it tolerated nothing like the contemporary American medical free-for-all. But, like Trudeau, Brehmer was a talented proselytizer and a skilled fund-raiser; he soon attracted influential adherents, including Alexander von Humboldt, who helped him clear a path through the formidable thickets of the relevant ministries. By the early 1850s Brehmer had raised a substantial sum of money, and, having finally secured the necessary government approval, he bought a 270-acre site in a mountain valley near Görbersdorf, a small Silesian hamlet a half hour from the nearest railway station, in the country southwest of Breslau. In 1859 the first building opened.

Whatever the weaknesses of Brehmer's theory, and despite his sister's thunderous shower-baths, his cook's Brobdingnagian meals, and his own orders for brisk mountain hikes, his patients, for whatever reason, flourished. Drawn by news of numerous and apparently absolute cures, they flocked to the sanatorium and it expanded rapidly. By 1880 it offered accommodations for 233 patients and had already spawned a number of European imitators, becoming a tourist destination as well as a health resort. Brehmer had, in a pattern to be repeated often in the next fifty years, constructed not merely a hospital but an enormous complex: "a huge Gothic pile," an admirer called it, "with towers, turrets and arches, consisting of three buildings of different dates, united in one line by covered passages and glazed galleries forming the winter garden."

One approached the hospital along "a murmuring rivulet of crystal purity," then found oneself stunned by the prospect of an "imposing palatial edifice" rearing out of the forest. "We are irresistibly reminded of one of those fairy palaces constructed by benevolent spirits in the course of a single night for the delight of some favoured mortal." The Kurhaus, the main building, a 460-foot-long Gothick extravaganza, consisted of two dining rooms, a reading room emblazoned with the arms of the countries from which patients hailed and equipped with a stage for theatrical performances; there were sitting rooms, verandas, and a Winter Garden planted with exotic blooms.

The grand staircase was a great vaulted cavern adorned with frescoes and "useful maxims" and furnished with alcoves where weaker patients could pause to rest. The rooms, "naturally varying in size . . . [present] every comfort that can be desired for an invalid."

The grounds were a marriage of nature and art, planned with a fanatical attention to detail that might be called Prussian if it weren't fated to be copied in other sanatoriums throughout Europe and the United States. There were walkways designed to match the capabilities of the patients. Benches were placed at strategic intervals, and small rest pavilions dotted the terrain. There were flower beds, shade trees, grottoes, mountain views, a trout pond, a statue of Asclepius, and a miniature temple containing a bust of Alexander von Humboldt. The sanatorium had its own model dairy farm, a separate brick and sandstone bathhouse for the shower treatments, and a carriage drive. Perched in the middle of it all, convenient to the Kurhaus, separated from it but easily accessible, was Brehmer's private residence, from which he supervised the intricate workings of a health resort that was halfway to becoming a private empire.

Brehmer's theories—exercise, food, and showers—were not the lasting part of his contribution to the antituberculosis movement. His pupil, and his first and most influential imitator, Peter Dettweiler, followed him in building a sanatorium (it opened at Falkenstein, in the Taunus Mountains, northwest of Frankfurt, in 1876), but grounded it on exactly opposite principles: Dettweiler's patients rested, avoiding all unnecessary exercise, and by 1900 the sanatorium movement had universally rejected Brehmer's regimen in favor of a modified version of Dettweiler's. But Brehmer had, in building Görbersdorf, tapped currents deeper and more profoundly influential than any system of specific therapies could possibly have touched. For he gave impressive embodiment to a belief nearly universal since the time of the Romantics in the healing power of landscapes, the wilder and more "natural" the better. Before the nineteenth century, for example, mountains had been thought of, when thought of at all, as horrid places, ugly, barren, dangerous, and unfit for humans; even the American Indians, otherwise intrepid, thought gods lived in them and wisely steered clear of them.

But with Goethe and his imitators, the spirit shifted; wild country in general and mountainscapes in particular became resorts of freedom, health, grandeur, and uplift. Your environment, as Henry Bowditch had explicitly argued in his *Atlantic* articles, had the power to make you well or ill; the grander the landscape the stronger its effect on the health. When, in "Tintern Abbey," Wordsworth described the valley view of the poem as producing even in memory sensations "felt in the blood, and felt along the heart," he was voicing a Romantic commonplace that scenery was not simply a background but an active force within the body of the observer. The belief soon spread to an important segment of the medical profession. *The English Practitioner*, for example, an influential and widely circulated English medical journal founded by Richard Anstey in 1868, included in virtually every issue throughout the 1870s and early 1880s various reports on the beneficial effects of different environments and different climates on disease. Over those years, South Africa, Tahiti, and the mountains of Peru all found advocates in the pages of the journal as locales beneficial for the consumptive; it was in the *Practitioner*, according to Trudeau, that he first read a description of the virtues of Brehmer's Görbersdorf establishment, and conceived the idea of imitating it in the Adirondacks.

That Brehmer decided to call his hospital a "sanatorium" illustrates the degree to which the power of place over body had become an article of medical faith. He dubbed Görbersdorf a *Heilanstalt*, or "healing institution." "San*i*ta rium," derived from the Latin word meaning "health," denotes, strictly speaking, only "a healthy place"; the term thus implies no curative effect. "Sana*to*rium," on the other hand, derives from "sanare," meaning "to heal," and thus means "a place of healing," a more accurate rendition of Brehmer's word. The American antituberculosis crusade enthusiastically endorsed the distinction; to use the term "sanitarium" became either an insult or a badge of ignorance about the movement. Even when it became plain that tuberculosis could effectively be cured in any landscape or climate (the point was proved by Vincent Bowditch—Henry's son—who in 1891 built a successful sanatorium in Sharon, Massachusetts, just outside Boston), the sanatorium movement never lost its conviction that the hospital's environment, man-made if not natural, was a vital factor in its success or failure.

That was one of Brehmer's legacies to the later history of the tuberculosis hospital, but there was another as well, perhaps even more pervasive. Romantically wild though Görbersdorf may have appeared to the casual observer, it was in fact a monument to foresight. Brehmer distinguished himself not only by the minuteness with which he designed his buildings and grounds but as well by the obsessive care with which he supervised his patients. Every moment of one's day was planned; walks were regulated to the inch; meal plans were subject to Brehmer's approval. The patient found every need anticipated, every exigency forestalled. And although the kinds of activities the sanatorium managed were to change over the next half century, the *principle* of management in every detail was to persist, at times in fact to run riot. There had been tuberculosis hospitals and health resorts before Brehmer's, but none so effectively combined a faith in the restorative powers of place with a devotion to the healing capabilities of minutely planned routine. And it was from these perhaps oddly paired twin ideologies that the American sanatorium movement was to rise.

In America the seeds of Brehmer's inspriation (and of Dettweiler's refinement of it) fell on fertile ground, appealing to a middle- and upper-class obsession with the wilderness. It was not only the heritage of the Romantics but disturbing statistics from the city slums that fed their conviction that the forests and mountains were a temple of health, a refuge from and a solution to the physical and moral evils of the town. Further, the return to the wilderness called up not merely vague emotional longing but a still fresh and influential memory of the earlier years of the republic when life was arranged wisely and simply in towns that were little more than villages.

In 1868 the Reverend William H. H. Murray of Boston had written *Adventures in the Wilderness; or, Camp-Life in the Adirondacks,* and launched an enduring fad for the region, an appreciation of its beauties, physical, moral, and medical. Later, in 1886, Joseph W. Stickler, M.D., published *The Adirondacks as a Health Resort.* The subject was, ostensibly, the beneficial effects of the climate there on consumptives, but, foreshadowing the sanatorium movement's later strong emphasis on character building, the contributors to the volume devote much attention to the region's moral advantages as a place suited to the battle against all the consequences of the Fall, not disease alone. The Reverend J. J. Duryea's essay, or rather homily, enumerated the antitubercular virtues of the Adirondacks and began with the purity and bracing temperature of the air, the cleanness of the water, the novelty of the landscape, and its blessed silence, as tonics for the depressed spirits of the consumptive. But he quickly rises to the advantages of "Seclusion from Temptation to Harmful Indulgence":

> The region has no population able and disposed to maintain means and methods of dissipation. Food is simple. Luxuries are costly, on account of freight. There are no "soda" fountains, ice-cream saloons, restaurants; lobsters are not to be found, to be mangled up with wilted lettuce, and soused with an infernal mixture out of a bottle. Melons do not abound. Dinner parties are not given.

At least during its early years, it is plain that Trudeau's fledgling Adirondack Cottage Sanatorium followed Brehmer and Dettweiler in this broad, philosophical spirit—Trudeau resisted adopting their sectarian medical regimens wholesale. His early patients, in the 1880s and 1890s, did rest, did take exercise, and did eat well, but not according to any rigid system. Like Dr. Stickler and the Reverend Duryea, Trudeau was convinced in a general way of the healing powers of the wilderness and seems not to have felt the need to translate this conviction into method.

His most famous experiment, conducted in 1885, illustrates the way his mind was working at the time. "I began to wonder how, if the tubercle bacillus had already gained access to the body, a change of climate, rest, fresh air and food could influence the disease." So he inoculated five rabbits with the tubercle bacillus and "turned them loose on a little island where they ran wild all summer in fresh air and sunshine, and had abundant food. All but one recovered and survived." Another lot of five less lucky rabbits, similarly inoculated, were put into "the worst environment I could devise—a dark, damp place where the air was bad, confined in a small box and fed insufficiently." Four of them were dead of tuberculosis within three months. The experiment would not hold up under modern scientific scrutiny (the numbers of animals were too small and the conditions to which they were subjected insufficiently controlled), but it became a famous rallying story in the antituberculosis movement, and it reveals the uniquely American twist Trudeau had given to the Brehmer model. Theory, albeit misguided, had given way to imaginative faith in the wilderness and freedom, albeit modified by some scientific skepticism. There had been a number of American tuberculosis hospitals, and at least one sanatorium,* before Trudeau's, but only his struck a note at once so resonant and so adaptable. Of *course* the free rabbits must flourish while the penned-up languish; fresh air, sunlight, good food, wholesome surroundings were appealing specifics that might be adapted to any number of therapeutic regimens, and throughout his career, Trudeau was to experiment with many.

But the cure in America was not to remain where Trudeau left it; in its heyday, between roughly 1910 and 1945, though

*The Channing Home in Boston had opened in 1857, as a refuge for tubercular women; in 1875 Joseph William Gleitsmann, a Bavarian physician, founded the Mountain Sanitarium for Pulmonary Diseases at Asheville, N.C. Little is known about this institution, which appears to have closed by 1880, except that patients spent much of their time in the open air and downed substantial meals prepared by Mrs. Gleitsmann.

it retained the mythic underpinnings Trudeau had given it in adapting it to American soil, it became much more widely publicized and far more systematic. These developments were collective and national in scope, for the movement was growing by leaps and bounds, and by 1910 could claim hundreds of influential figures. But two stand out: Lawrason Brown and S. Adolphus Knopf. A generation younger than Trudeau and Alfred Loomis, they yet recalled the partnership that made the latter pair such a potent force; for Brown, working more or less obscurely in Saranac Lake, turned the cure from a relatively informal routine to a minutely calibrated system of rest, exercise, and diet, while Knopf, based in New York, indefatigably proselytized, publicizing the cure in particular and the movement in general. Their respective books, Brown's *Rules for Recovery from Pulmonary Tuberculosis* (1916) and Knopf's *Tuberculosis as a Disease of the Masses and How to Combat It* (first published in 1899 and much reprinted), became classics in the War on Consumption, and between them helped define for at least two generations the way sanatoriums were run and the ways the public perceived them.

They were a contrasting pair. Brown had become resident physician at the Adirondack Cottage Sanatorium in 1901 and remained there until 1912, refining and systematizing the treatment patients underwent, formulating rules, and governing the minutest details of their days. Thereafter he left the sanatorium and set up a private practice in Saranac Lake, though retaining his affiliation with Trudeau; he was to become a fixture, even an institution, in the village. He is remembered as an owlish, taciturn, and rather untidy figure; plagued by foot trouble, he used to shuffle in bedroom slippers through the streets and into the sickrooms of his patients, on whom, however unprepossessing his appearance, he had an uplifting effect. "He's swell," Marshall McClintock, a Saranac patient in the 1920s, recalled telling his wife. "I always feel so damned healthy for days after he has been here." He was also charitable, treating large numbers of impoverished patients for free, and, despite his apparently successful bedside manner, scholarly, with a passion for organization. The Trudeau Institute retains one of his typescripts, "A Tuberculosis Chronology," an elaborate digest history of the disease, crammed with facts, and arranged systematically from 5000 B.C. to 1931.

Knopf cut in every way a different figure; voluble, public, and excitable where Brown was silent, inward, and methodical. While Brown largely stayed put in Saranac, Knopf traveled everywhere, becoming the most widely known and vocal public authority on tuberculosis. Born and raised in Prussia, with its long-established tradition of enlightened and systematized medical care, Knopf crusaded against what he dubbed "phthisophobia," or the irrational fear of the disease and its victims. An intense figure, with brisk mustache and goatee, much at pains to improve the medical care in his adopted country (he was, understandably, particularly eager to declare his patriotism during World War I), he gave brisk public lectures, wrote blistering letters to the editors of newspapers guilty of misleading articles on tuberculosis. He was an energetic apostle of cold baths, a declared enemy of girdles and other confining garments, and an inventor, among other things, of the Knopf-Thibert Elevated Self-Flushing Spittoon. His pamphlets blanketed the nation throughout the public hygiene–conscious 1920s.

The great, overarching theme of the heyday of the tuberculosis cure, as Brown formulated it and Knopf publicized it, was the Outdoor Life. By 1916, when Brown wrote *Rules for Recovery from Pulmonary Tuberculosis*, rest had in fact become the dominant factor in sanatorium routine, replacing exercise, which was allowed in increasing doses only as the patient edged toward normal life. But inactivity, crucial though it was in the sanatorium, implied passivity and helplessness. Resting outdoors, day and night, summer and winter, made rest into a challenge, and almost into a cult. Brown, observing that most patients gained weight at the Adirondack Cottage Sanatorium from August through December, remained stationary through spring, then again lost weight steadily through August, reasoned that this was brought about by the abrupt seasonal changes in the Adirondacks and that the fluctuation must be a tonic. He insisted on maximizing the patient's exposure to the open air and to shifts in weather, even in midwinter. The patient who sat inside was " 'unfaithful to the cure'—that is, stay-in when he should be out—he is retarding his recovery and inviting more serious illness. . . . He should develop an 'outdoor conscience.' " Of course, fresh air had been a preoccupation of doctors for decades, but the sanatorium made it into a vocation, a craft with its own repertory of techniques, and governed by rules. Typically, instructions were given to every patient upon admission; the Massachusetts State Sanatorium at Rutland was characteristic: "Patients must spend as much time as possible out of doors every day. They must be out of the wards before nine A.M."

Knopf joined Brown in this obsession, and in fact rather intensified it. "It is surprising," he wrote,

> how easily consumptives get accustomed to the pro-longed sojourn in the open air. Neither change of weather, cold, rain, snow, nor even wind, providing it is not too strong, hinders the patients from spending most of their time on the piazza, porch, or rest cure gallery. . . . Dr. Andvord, of the Tonsaasen Sanatorium, reported that his patients remained in the open air from five to nine hours a day at a temperature of 13°F. below zero, and felt very well. Similiar [sic] reports come to us from that excellent American institution, the Adirondack Cottage Sanatorium, under the direction of Dr. Edward L. Trudeau, the pioneer of the sanatorium treatment in the United States. We reproduce a photograph (Fig. 19) taken on a winter day at that institution, showing how well and comfortable the patients are in spite of the cold. We also give a typical German rest-cure gallery or "Liegehalle" (Fig. 20) and finally a picture representing the rest cure in the summer in the woods at a sanatorium in the Black Forest in Germany (Fig. 21). The latter shows how the patients in a sanatorium know how to have a good time.

In fact, the inmates in all three photographs look immobile and rather wretched. Like Brown, Knopf is unable to specify, except vaguely, how fresh air helps the consumptive; rather he devotes his arguments to proving it harmless and easy for the patients to endure. Its beneficial effects were taken for granted, swallowed uncritically as myth, even by physicians who were, in bacteriological matters, hardheaded empiricists. Initially Brehmer's sanatorium operated only in the summer, not admitting patients for a winter cure until 1862; the idea that fresh air helped the disease grew out of the sanatorium movement rather than spawning it.

Yet once it took root, this enthusiasm was to persist, though it was emphasized less strenuously as time went on. It was worked into the physical design of sanatorium buildings and became, whatever its clinical merits, a rallying point. And no doubt it had some value. Sitting out in the cold helped alleviate some of the tedium of the rest cure. Although it immobilized you underneath layers of rugs and blankets (any movement let in freezing air) it also confronted you with a challenge, made you feel you were facing down the elements, living with a vitality and a pioneering spirit unknown to the dwellers in the overheated rooms of the city.

Sanatorium advocates routinely praised the Outdoor Life as an antidote to the moral, spiritual, and physical ills of urban crowding. The decor Knopf prescribes for the invalid's room is as much a rebellion against Victorian tastes in furniture as a prescription for health. "Plush velvet or cloth covered furniture, heavy curtains or other fancy decorations, which might serve as dust-catchers, should not be allowed in the room of a tuberculous patient. Leather-covered, rattan, and plain wooden furniture are certainly the best and the curtains should always be of washable material." The fad for fresh air revealed, in other words, an underlying impatience with the overdressed, overupholstered, overheated, and overdecorated tastes of the nineteenth century, at least as partisans of the Outdoor Life saw them. It was not merely their lungs that the tuberculous were being asked to open to the country breezes but also the rooms they dwelt in and even their bodies. And in so doing, patients were counseled to follow explicit directions.

Indeed, detailed instructions were introduced about everything from the way patients were to inhale the outdoor air to
the lounge equipment and bodily positions they used to ingest
it. The first weeks of the invalid's stay in the sanatorium served
as both an orientation and an indoctrination in "right living."

The instructions, of course, inevitably varied from authority
to authority, but were always uncompromisingly detailed. The
cure porch, Lawrason Brown wrote, "should face south by
southwest in winter and north in summer, but a southern
porch shaded well in summer by deciduous trees is usually
very habitable." For the rest hours he recommended the Adi-
rondack-style chair, a frame contraption with a movable back
and an adjustable footrest, and a small industry grew up in
Saranac Lake to supply them. The chair, in turn, couldn't be
used haphazardly; Brown provided detailed instructions for
how to wrap oneself up before lying in it.

> Place the rug, which should be large in size, fully ex-
> tended on the chair. After sitting down grasp the part of
> the rug lying on the right of the chair and with a quick
> motion throw it over the feet and knees and tuck it well
> under the legs. Then do the same with the part of the rug
> on the other side of the chair but leave the edge free. Now
> grasp the free edge of the rug lying on the right hand side
> and pull it up hand over hand until the end which was
> lying free beyond the feet is reached. Then pull up the far
> end of the rug, taking care to uncover as little as possible
> of the legs, and tuck both sides under the knees. This will
> give three or four layers of rug over most of the legs but
> only one over the feet. It forms, however, a bag out of the
> rug and no air can enter. A second rug folded and thrown
> over the first makes such a covering that the coldest
> weather can be defied.

Tuberculosis was at best an unpredictable disease. Diagnosis
was, and to a degree still is, uncertain. Its grosser symptoms
could be mistaken for other, less serious illnesses; X rays were
often ambiguous. Even a positive skin test meant only that you
had been exposed to the disease, not that you had a clinical
case of it. Once a diagnosis was made, the prognosis was

equally uncertain: the memoirs of patients and the medical literature are full of gradual improvements, sudden setbacks, miraculous recoveries, and unexpected relapses. The emphasis on method was thus a reaction to this uncertainty. System in the sanatorium was not so much a direct treatment as a giant, living metaphor of order, erected in the face of the unpredictable, as a bulwark against it.

This extended from the use of the cure chair and instructions for proper breathing and dressing to the layout of the patient's day, week, and year. Tuberculosis was always slow in the controlling, and sanatorium stays of upward of twenty years were not unheard of, so that time could become almost as daunting and unmanageable as the ebb and flow of the illness itself. As a result the simplest events of daily life took on a therapeutic importance and became invested with the superstition of ritual.

Lawrason Brown gives a typical regimen for the patient's day:

7:30	Awake. Take temperature. Milk (hot if desired) if necessary.
	Warm water for washing. Cold sponge.
8:00	Breakfast
8:30	Out of doors in chair or on bed
10:30	Lunch when ordered
11–1	Exercise or rest as ordered
1–2	Dinner. Indoors not over one hour, less if possible.
2–4	Rest in reclining position. Reading, but no talking allowed.
	Take temperature.
3:30	Lunch when ordered.
4–6	Exercise in prescribed amount.
6:00	Supper
7:00	Out on good nights
8:00	Take temperature.
9:00	Lunch and bed.

The hours are the hours of childhood; the day is divided into contrasting blocks of time, rest, exercise, eating, punctuated three times by temperature taking (although not all prescribed this so frequently). The daily plan varied only once or twice weekly, with a hot bath followed by a cold sponge. In the latter practice Brown was comparatively conservative: Knopf thought forty degrees an ideal temperature for the bathwater, and remained influential in this matter through the 1920s. He recommended a gradual acclimation to the freezing plunge, however: the patient was introduced to it by an alcohol rub for the first few days, the alcohol then replaced by sponging with colder and colder water.

Some hospitals were more strict than Brown recommended. Absolute silence might be enforced during all rest periods, particularly during the early stages of the cure—Betty Mac-Donald's Seattle sanatorium forbade its female patients to read during the early weeks of the treatment. But all were committed to order in the day not just as a convenience for the staff or a necessary economy in the running of a large institution but as a benefit in its own right. With the early rising, the early retiring, the moderate use of rest, activity, and eating, the sanatorium was battling tuberculosis: this was the mainspring of its medical theory, to which medication and surgical intervention always took a back seat. It was not really scientific; individual patient behavior, hospital routines, and admission policies (many sanatoriums refused to accept advanced cases) made it impossible ever to determine how much better sanatorium patients did than those who tried to follow the cure at home. But in the years before surgery became commonplace, it convinced patients of its wholesomeness and effectiveness intuitively, by the simple device of codifying folk convictions about what was healthy. It was simply a medical institutionalizing of advice Poor Richard might have given; a therapeutic exaggeration of a normal healthy day.

This is nowhere clearer than in the matter of meals. Brehmer's Rabelaisian repasts had largely (though not entirely) fallen out of fashion by the early twentieth century, but carefully controlled eating remained, on a more moderate scale, a central feature of the cure and a focus of the day, as carefully supervised by the institution as the Outdoor Life. Until they closed down in the 1950s, virtually all sanatoriums prided themselves on serving food well above the abysmal hospital average. Good food built the body and kept the spirits up. And, particularly earlier in the century, the idea prevailed that a fortifying diet was a powerful specific against consumption. Though it later became the orthodox view that overeating taxed the system and hence took its toll on the lungs, the brief for enthusiastic eating had an intuitive attraction: If the disease devours one, what better way to battle it than to outpace in your own consumption of food the disease in its consumption of you? You were in a race with tuberculosis, and with luck and application you might out-consume it.

Not surprisingly, then, the salaries paid, on the average, to sanatorium employees reflects the centrality of food to the cure. In his influential book on sanatorium planning Thomas S. Carrington, M.D., suggested $2,500 per annum for the physician director of the hospital, $1,200 for his assistant, and $600 for a laboratory director (both of the latter also physicians). Nurses, apparently expected to devote themselves selflessly to the service of their patients, were paid, in the spirit of self-sacrifice, a Dickensian $180 per year each—barely more than half the $300 per year given to orderlies. (Though Carrington does not so specify, it may be that he expected nurses to live at the hospital, and hence to be spared the expense of room and board.)

But the dietitian was to be paid $900 per year, the cook $960, the gardener and baker $720 each—all more than the laboratory director earned, little less than the assisting physician, and four times as much as the nurses. Even waitresses and maids, at $216 per year, fared better. The relative salaries accorded different personnel are mirrored in their relative numbers: a sanatorium for 100 patients would, in Carrington's estimation, employ fifty-one people. Of these, eighteen, or more than a third, would be engaged in the production, preparation, or serving of food.

"It is an old adage among patients of tuberculosis," Lawrason Brown wrote, "that they should eat once for themselves, once for the germs, and once to gain weight." Eating was medicinal, and the preparation of the invalid's diet became a matter not merely of feeding but of preparing foods as if they were pharmacological compounds, calibrating ingredients and dosages precisely. Charles Fox Gardiner, author of *The Care of the Consumptive* (1900), prescribed a typical diet, more moderate than those advocated by many authorities, but robust by modern standards. On awakening, the patient was to drink a half pint of milk and eat a piece of toast ("in making toast, use stale bread, cut thin, and toast quickly"). Breakfast, less than an hour later, should include eggs (poached, soft-boiled, or raw), mutton chops or broiled steak, poultry, sweetbreads, scraped raw meat, sardines ("if found digestible"), crisp bacon, "mush of several kinds provided it is boiled at least four hours," fruit (though "pineapples, bananas, and all tropical fruits are not allowed"), and bread (two days old). "The food must be eaten slowly; imperfect teeth should be attended to in order that the food may be properly masticated."

Dinner, at noon, was a heartier version of breakfast: "roast beef, mutton, turkey; vegetables—baked potatoes, for instance, or well-boiled spinach, easily digested peas, corn, cauliflower, lettuce with lemon juice; game, such as boiled or roasted partridge, squab, woodcock, snipe, prairie chicken, or quail; and, as a vegetable substitute, macaroni or spaghetti, cooked without cheese; some light pudding, such as rice or bread pudding or that made from stewed fruits; ice cream (taken with caution)." A lunch, at 4:00 P.M., might include "milk toast, scraped meat, or a cup of milk; bouillion, crackers or zwieback; cocoa, beef juice, milk punch or egg-nogg; raw egg, broth, or a few raw oysters; possibly tea with a dash of rum; and sandwiches made with jelly or Dundee marmalade, or English breakfast biscuits. Panopeptone is useful." Supper, served between six and eight, should include "tropon stirred into milk or broth; cold meats or warm chops or steak; broiled fish or trout; no canned foods of any sorts, except sardines."

Dr. Gardiner's patients would have required a farm to feed them; but he was, for his time, not excessive, particularly in his emphasis on protein, and more particularly in his insistence on the importance of milk and eggs (this receded in the 1930s). Yet it is not so much the specifics of his diet as the fact of their existence—the air of authority with which foods are recommended, the conviction that every dish is the product of calculation, selected for a reason, as if one scoop of ice cream too many or one sardine too few might ruin the health-giving properties of the diet. Why no canned foods save sardines? Why boil breakfast mush for four hours? Why must bread be two days old? What, come four o'clock, is the rationale behind a snack of raw oysters and jelly sandwiches?

Only that everything was measured—the food, the times for rest and activity, and the patient himself. And that everything mattered. Patient temperatures were taken in all sanatoriums at least once a day: a gradual return from fever to normal was a sign of improvement. Weights, over the long run perhaps the most crucial and substantial index of progress or decline, were typically taken once a week, and could be the most exhilarating or the most traumatic of the sanatorium rituals. Patients were of course also subjected to periodic X rays and other forms of examination, but they understandably remembered the weigh-ins with particular vividness. In his 1921 play *The Straw,* Eugene O'Neill—himself veteran of a short stay at the Gaylord Farm Sanatorium in Wallingford, Connecticut—devoted an entire scene to the ritual. As his failing heroine, Eileen Carmody, mounts the scale and receives the bad news of a further setback, even O'Neill's stage directions capture the tension of the moment and its importance as a dramatic break in the supposed monotony of hospital life.

Eventually a patient who kept losing weight, whose X rays failed to show improvement, whose sputum revealed the continuing presence of tubercle bacilli, whose weight decreased or whose temperature refused to stabilize might be sent to the sanatorium's infirmary and be subjected to a more rigid routine, or more radical forms of treatment like surgery. But the infirmary was rarely spoken about; and often it was regarded by ambulent patients with dread. The accepted model was slow but steady improvement, measured against the stable rituals of the cure.

The sanatoriums, already regulating their patients' rest ("Rest," according to the Metropolitan Life Insurance Company facility at Mount McGregor, meant "complete relaxation of body and mind. You are not relaxed if you lie with your arms behind your head, read or listen to the radio."), their activity, their food ("always drink milk slowly" and never discuss disease or symptoms, "especially during meals. Digestion is aided by a pleasant atmosphere."), and the fluctuations in their bodies, naturally also planned their intellectual pursuits. There were rule books—every patient received one upon entry to every institution—and there were forms. The Barlow Sanatorium in California had a packet assigned to every patient including temperature charts, records of physical examinations, and other details.

Most sanatoriums also published in-house magazines, ranging from mimeographed broadsheets like "Stony Wold Sez" at the Stony Wold Sanatorium near Saranac Lake, to professionally printed journals like Mount McGregor's *Optimist;* patients could also subscribe to *Journal of the Outdoor Life,* the sanatorium patients' national magazine founded by Lawrason Brown. On special occasions, like the fifteenth anniversary of the Gaylord Farm Sanatorium, they could look forward to addresses from luminaries like S. Adolphus Knopf.

All these media had one thing in common: a fondness, bordering on a mania, for maxims. Doctors used them to encourage patients as they convalesced, and sometimes to browbeat them if they rebelled. Maxims and proverbs educated people about the cure. More subtly, proverbs are traditionally epigrams about how to get through normal life, and perhaps their presence made the hospital seem less an exile colony, and more a part of the life going on outside it. Why else the persistent emphasis in such epigrams on work, striving, and effort?

Some Aphorisms for the Tuberculosis Patient

1.   "The labor which best repays a sick man is to get well."

2.   "Desire but one thing" (to get well) "and that with all thy heart."

3.   "Whatever thou takest in hand remember the end, and thou shalt never do amiss."

4.   "Whatever is worth doing is worth doing well."

9.   "Be intent only on that which thou art now doing and on the instrument by which thou doest it."

10.   "Your most important duty is to get well. Let all other duties be secondary."

Implicitly, the fate of the body depends on the mind; a sanatorium spent as much of its effort drumming this idea into its patients as it did intervening in their bodies.

If one progressed satisfactorily, inactivity gradually gave way to exercise. By Lawrason Brown's advice this began with a daily trip to the toilet. Next, one was allowed to sit up in a chair, and when this had built up to two or three hours a day, one was allowed to dress oneself, then advance to level walking. But progress could be interrupted or reversed by the slightest sign of a bad reaction—temperature, weight loss, or even signs of a languishing mind. "A slight feeling of lassitude, slight loss of strength, a sense of fatigue from the accustomed exercise ('lack of ginger,' some would call it), the appetite loses its keenness, a disinclination to get up after two hours in bed, a slight headache"—all these were reasons for a return to complete bed rest. If the European founders of the modern sanatorium regimen had initially laid out opposite theories of exercise—Brehmer heartily approved of it, Dettweiler dethroned it in favor of rest—by the early twentieth century in America a solution had been reached in a careful apportioning between the two. The fine discriminations thought necessary in dividing them were to be made by the physician, a testament to his skill and intuition. The doctor knew, in theory, exactly how much rest and how much activity were right for you at each stage of the cure. If you were a good patient, you let him calibrate precisely every detail of your daily routine; every minute was lived by doctor's orders, and the result was tested by every ounce of weight gained or lost, every tenth of a degree of fever.

Knopf, that most redoubtable of all antituberculosis crusaders, trumpeted the ascendancy of the physician in a September 3, 1919, speech at Gaylord Farm, on the occasion of that institution's fifteenth anniversary. His topic was "The Ideal Sanatorium, the Ideal Physician, the Ideal Nurse, the Ideal Patient," and the speech itself a rousing affirmation of optimism. The sanatorium, Knopf argued in another theme to become ubiquitous in the movement, should not be thought of as a hospital or a hopeless resort for the fatally ill but "a school, a college where the patients can and must learn many things. . . . The physician is the teacher, the nurse is the assistant teacher, the patients are the pupils." The physician must know everything about each of his patients, because he is charged with integrating them smoothly into an ideal social community. "I wish Dr. Fishberg"—an authority who had, to Knopf's outrage, recently branded consumptives as constitutionally selfish—"could be here today to see this throng of patients and to look in their bright and happy faces where it would be difficult for him to discover a sign of selfishness because good friendship and perfect gratitude toward the sanatorium and their physician is plainly visible in every face." Similarly, according to Edward O. Otis, a doctor with a more than vested interest in the matter, nature demanded three things of the hopeful patient: first, constant control by the physician, then good food and "the constant and continuous exposure of the patient to pure outdoor air night and day," and finally "Tranquillity and hopefulness of mind, for the mental condition has much to do with the success of the treatment."

In the last analysis, as its advocates framed it, the Outdoor Life and its elaborate methodical appurtenances appealed, both to patients and doctors, not so much because of their effect on the lungs, which always remained debatable, but because the cure was a discipline, an affirmation of order and predictability in the face of pain, dissolution, chaos. Tuberculosis might not be cured (though an arrest of the disease process might be hoped for), but sanatorium life could throw up a small redoubt of system against an onslaught of destruction. Control, impossible to implement fully over the disease, therefore had to be applied to the patient and his life; therein lay the best hope for arrest.

In a pamphlet called *Gleanings from Twelve Years' Constant Residence in a Sanatorium for the Treatment of Pulmonary Tuberculosis*, M. J. Brooks, M.D., insisted on this:

> Consumption is curable in the majority of cases, provided that there is sincere and proper treatment. This can only be accomplished where the patients are under constant, competent, painstaking medical supervision under one roof. For there is no disease requiring more persistent care, more absolute, perfect control. Every detail of the patient's life should be under constant observation.

Brooks ran a private sanatorium in New Canaan, Connecticut, and this pamphlet was in effect an advertisement for it, designed to attract patients. The importance of control was thus not only a support for the physician's authority; it appears to have been a drawing card for the patient as well.

American sanatoriums forcefully expressed the philosophy of benevolent control espoused by Knopf, Otis, and Brooks. Design was standardized early in the movement, mainly by the National Tuberculosis Association but also by various government agencies that began to interest themselves in the building of public sanatoriums. *Tuberculosis Hospital and Sanatorium Construction*, by Thomas Carrington, was first published in 1911 by the National Association for the Study and Prevention of Tuberculosis and frequently revised and reissued thereafter. It became the bible of sanatorium planning.

It was highly specific, but its detail was firmly harnessed to a central principle: "It may . . . be said that those who adhere to simplicity and economy in sanatorium construction and furnishing, and who furnish patients with good wholesome food, cleanliness, light employment, and a happy, friendly atmosphere, are operating along modern and approved lines."

Yet frugality was important. In Europe, consumption had been thought a refined ailment, but in America it emerged in public awareness as a disease of the poor. Care for its victims became a public responsibility. The ill should be housed and fed well, but not luxuriously, and thus Brehmer's imposing pile gave way in the United States to an architecture of rustic simplicity. Carrington estimated that in 1914 an adequate sanatorium housing 100 patients could be built for between $38,000 and $63,000. Recommending, however, a more elaborate plan, he broke anticipated expenses down, and the division reveals perhaps as much about the psychological and social structure of the typical sanatorium as about its physical plant:

Administration Building	$31,500
4 lean-tos	14,000
2 wards for advanced cases	14,000
Power House and Heating Plant	5,000
Sewage disposal plant	2,000
Water pumping and supply plant	5,000
Boilers and machinery	3,300
Furnishings	7,000
Laundry	1,200
Land (site)	5,500
Building Commission Expenses	11,500

The large-ticket items are for what was most essential in the sanatorium ideology—control. Between them the administration building and the unspecified expenses of the building commission account for 43 percent of the total cost of the project. Accommodations for patients were, structurally, a low priority—all of them combined were to cost less than the administration building. Inevitably this meant that the administrative center dominated the sanatorium landscape, a natural consequence of the importance in the cure of supervising the patient's daily life. Always distinguished from the patient quarters by its central place in the plan, the administration building was built at least a story higher; Carrington, allowing patient cottages to be made of lightweight materials, nonetheless specified that the administration centers should be "constructed of substantial material on lines that can be enlarged when necessary." Cottages or dormitories simply multiplied; central buildings grew.

Carrington reflected the actual practice of the sanatoriums quite accurately. A typical example was the Maryland State Sanatorium at Sabillasville. Standing in the foreground and much the largest, the administration building suggests, both in its solidity and the luxury of its detail, a manor house. It is approached by a monumental stairway, whereas all the other buildings on the site are flush with the ground. It is the head of a body; the service building behind it receives orders from it and channels them to the patient cottages arrayed behind it. No doubt the architect did not design it on a conscious analogy with a head and a pair of lungs, but the similarity with a human body, even to the passageways that link the major organs, is striking.*

Two dominant sanatorium ground plans were to emerge. The cottage model pioneered and perhaps best exemplified by the Adirondack Cottage Sanatorium arrayed itself around a central administration building and infirmary. But bungalow-like accommodations for most patients, deliberately built to different designs, were scattered more or less informally throughout the grounds, and intended as far as was practical to be homelike. The institutional plan of which Sabillasville was typical arranged the patient accommodations differently, designing them more like hospital wards (though most often small ones, each with its own central living room) and connecting them formally to the administrative center via a network of corridors, covered walkways, or tunnels. But the relation

---

*This is still more the case with the design for the Georgia State Sanatorium at Alto, built on two spurs of a hill—its similarity to a pair of lungs is unmistakable. Interestingly enough, there is a separate hospital for black patients, built on the same overall plan, but with the patient cottages much closer to the supervision of the administration building.

between the central building and the satellite cottages or dormitories was always the same. The passion for central control suggests forcibly the town planning of ancient imperial cultures—Roman, Chinese, Aztec, Incan. Their towns all featured a central axis, flanked by dwellings and tributary structures, all leading formally to a site of dominant ceremonial importance, temple or administrative headquarters. These towns were designed to impress upon the populace the importance of the central power, whatever it was, and often to inspire as much dread as respect. The optimistic philosophy of the cure was, of course, supposed to banish dread; but one of the most persistent memories among ex-patients was a mortal fear of the administration building. More often than not it was also the site of the infirmary, hence a place to which you were sent if you suffered a relapse. And, of course, it suggested the New England town, ranged in orderly subjection to the church, which lent the central authority a traditional as well as an intimidating aura.

Sleeping cottages themselves, in the majority of sanatorium plans (the Adirondack Cottage Sanatorium was a major exception), were also designed according to the dominant ethic of centralization. Typically there was a central communal living room, backed by bathrooms and lockers for patients' belongings, and flanked by two long dormitories, each fronted by a porch. The "living" area and the patients' possessions are central, but they are also the smallest space in the complex. Resting areas, less central, are nonetheless more extensive, and ranged so as to permit the maximum possible supervision. The living room often had comfortable furniture, amusements, a heat source, even a fireplace; the sleeping quarters were rarely heated, had no nooks, merely beds arranged in stern rows, facing outdoors. Some were more elaborate than others, but sleeping dormitories were nearly always Spartan, particularly by contrast with the central facilities of the hospital. At times, as at the New York City municipal sanatorium at Otisville, New York, the dormitories were mere lean-tos; elsewhere they were more substantial but still simple.

Some American sanatoriums, of course, emulated the megalithic quality of European hospitals like Brehmer's: the Agnes Memorial Sanatorium at Denver was a characteristic example, far more a single institution than was typical, and showing little cellular division. But the cottage plan was the dominant force in American sanatorium design, even where it was only partially applied. The breaking down of accommodations into small, quasi-familial cells allowed for a sense of smallness, intimacy, communion with the outdoors. Americans wanted, it seems, to live in groups but were beginning to hate their choked cities; the sanatorium built on the cottage plan harked back to a time when the country was a place of small villages of manageable and unthreatening scale, fostering the independence of their citizens without leaving them unprotected. Yet woven in this tapestry of rural informality was a subtle but pervasive atmosphere of centralized power—the administration everywhere visible, with easy access to every cottage, often represented within the cottage itself by a nurses' station in or next to the living room. The sanatorium was a federal system, a model of the country it existed in, but from the social fabric of which it was largely isolated.

As sanatoriums multiplied and the movement matured, it became a source of national pride. In 1885 the nation had only Trudeau's Little Red, with a mere two female patients; by 1935 there were, according to the American Medical Association, 471 full-fledged sanatoriums in the nation, and 418 more tuberculosis departments connected with general hospitals; in that same year there were 95,198 beds available for the treatment of tuberculosis. The more forward-looking states had elaborate public sanatorium systems: by 1920 New York had required every county in the state to build and maintain a sanatorium for its citizens. Enlightened mercantile interests (or at least those wanting to be perceived as enlightened) like Metropolitan Life and the Standard Oil Company (which persuaded the Loomis Sanatorium in upstate New York to erect a building devoted exclusively to the treatment of its tubercular employees) also became involved in the movement.

What was emerging in these years, only to fade as the morbidity rate from the disease sank and the biological weapons against it rendered it controllable, was an ad hoc system of socialized medicine, an improvised but nonetheless cohesive system, based on cooperation among government, private enterprise, organized medicine, and simple community spirit. Early in its history de Tocqueville had noted America's passion for voluntary associations—informal groupings of citizens in support of a cause, which, bonding together, used the power of the press to engender awareness of their concerns and turn themselves into an effective social force. The sanatorium movement was preeminently such an association, on an unprecedented national scale, and not duplicated since.

Of course Standard Oil, New York State, and Carrington's national association meant well by their employees, citizens, and beneficiaries. But the attraction of such different interests—corporate, governmental, and voluntary—toward a single goal has another dimension, particularly when one considers the power in the sanatorium movement of the idea of central control. Remarks made by Dr. James Miller of New York and Seth B. Hunt of Standard Oil at the 1896 dedication of the Loomis pavilion bear this out. Miller envisioned "the beginning of a broad movement among commercial enterprises to . . . care for their employees by the maintenance of systematic medical inspection and treatment." Hunt was more explicit still:

> The building of this cottage where employees of the Standard Oil Company (New Jersey) who unfortunately have tuberculosis can cure, is really a logical result of a plan introduced by our Company something over three years ago. In this plan, beside arranging for industrial relations, we considered particularly the three serious problems that all of us face . . . illness, old age, and death.

In taking on such challenges, according to Hunt, Standard Oil was showing the American way as superior to "the experiments that have been made abroad in England and some of the

European countries, where the government bears this expense in the shape of old-age pensions, doles, etc." Hunt and Standard Oil prefer the voluntary approach:

> While the community as a whole can only care for the advanced cases of tuberculosis, the employer, with his closer relation to the wage-earner, can readily detect early cases, when good treatment so often promises recovery, and when the removal of contagion saves others, both in the industry and the families.

Central control thus speaks in the language of democracy; or perhaps democracy simply reveals its inner nature as a mode of control. Yet the cottage plan was more than a device for the exercise of power. Informality and humbleness seemed natural to patients whose means were at best modest, and did not oppress them with unaccustomed and unnecessary luxury, rendering them malcontents when they got home. Carrington had forcefully advised that cottages be built as inexpensively as possible, because "this class of institution returns patients to their homes without making them unduly discontented with the environment and life to which they belong."

Small comforts were allowed, but not carried too far; normal life was imitated, but not lived. The sexes were separated, except for carefully supervised occasions and at limited times. Personal possessions were kept in lockers, away from patient beds, and subjected to the examination and the ministrations of the staff. "As it is undesirable to have bags and boxes in the bedrooms, cupboards or wardrobes of some kind are necessary. . . . The chief objection to their presence is that they may escape the daily cleaning which is so important for every part of the room." Mystery and complexity are banished from the patient's life; they are unclean and inappropriate to the rusticity of the cure.

In their enthusiasm for planning, their insistence that everything in the life of the sanatorium should serve efficiently the regimen of the cure, the leaders of the movement may have been exercising power over the lives of the humble. But they were also reflecting a general current of enthusiasm in the late nineteenth and early twentieth centuries for town plans that were in feeling as much countrified as urban, organized, but full of open vistas and imitations of rural space.

The practical Carrington reflects this in his specifications for sanatorium design. The land, he argued, should be a microcosm, comprehending every sort of terrain in miniature: forest, orchard, open land capable of cultivation. In an extension of Brehmer's scrupulous design, Carrington argued that the sanatorium should be self-contained and if possible completely self-supporting, with the completeness of a town in the openness of the countryside. Apart from the administration building and patient cottages, Carrington demands a complete working farm, with greenhouses and cold frames, a milk house, barns for cows, hogs, and horses. But rural pursuits should be supplemented by the means for industry: Carrington prescribed an industrial building as well, with facilities for "light carpentering, cabinetmaking, taxidermy, art work, . . . photography," and, in the spirit of medical as well as economic self-sufficiency, "a machine for stamping out sputum cups." There should be a bakery, an icehouse, an amusement pavilion, laundry, post office, railroad station, and a telephone exchange.

In short a model city planted in the heart of the country, a philanthropic gesture toward the well-being of the sick, but a paradigm as well of commercial development for rural areas: "The sanatorium has a great educational value; it gives employment to local people; it has a payroll of from $1,000 to $1,500 per month, a part of which, at least, is expended in the neighborhood; it brings friends and visitors to nearby hotels; benefits the merchants; and creates a market for produce raised in the vicinity." Illness, therefore, need not be only a disaster for the ill; it can form the basis of an economy.

The difference, in other words, between the hospital and the sanatorium was the difference between a narrowly conceived technological mechanism designed to deliver specialized medical services efficiently, and a full-blown ideology. Sanatorium planning paralleled a widespread interest in late-nineteenth-century America in ideal planned communities. John Humphrey Noyes, the founder of the Oneida Community, perhaps the best known, grounded his experiment on a doctrine he called Perfectionism: human life, Noyes thought, lived communally and with determined simplicity, could be perfect, if controlled by a leader who supervised every aspect of the community's physical, economic, and spiritual life. Improper communal living, he charged, was the root cause of both physical weakness and illness.

The Chautauqua movement, begun by the Reverend John Heyl Vincent and Lewis Miller in 1874 (roughly the same time as the sanatorium movement got under way), reflects the same spirit. Vincent and Miller's aim was neither to found a utopia nor cure a disease but to train Sunday School teachers in an attractive camplike setting by Chautauqua Lake, in the southwest corner of New York State. But their project burgeoned, attracted thousands, expanded in scope, and became a national educational movement. Every summer people from all walks of life descended on the site, which grew into a bizarre combination of a college campus and a revivalist camp meeting. The students lived and ate simply, enjoyed simple recreations like swimming in the lake, and attended lectures, concerts, and classes. The combination of informal outdoor living, social interaction, and self-improvement struck a major chord in the American psyche, appealing to an apparent hunger for education stripped of the intimidating and class-bound trappings of the country's better known schools and colleges. The informality and democratism of the movement was appealing; so too was the firm control of an authority figure who presided over it: teachers at Chautauqua were revered and lived separately from and better than their students.

All such ideal communities, whether sanatorium or rural utopia, had in common the desire to impose control on the chaos of experience while retaining at least the semblance of democracy; they used the countryside to arouse soothing images of freedom and escape, while organizing within themselves an urban complex of networks and hierarchies. Perhaps the antituberculosis movement had the best rationale for this, as it set itself against more than merely philosophical terrors— its enemy was not merely disorganization but death. Passively giving up power over your own life when you entered, you were told, and apparently often believed, that you were embarking on a battle that would demand all your reserves of energy and determination. Lying flat on your back, you were in training to be a conqueror. Submitting your smallest action to the control of a rule book, patiently observing the routine, you were temporarily sacrificing your independence in the hopes of regaining it and holding it more firmly than you had before. The American sanatorium took the two apparently opposing themes first sounded by Brehmer and Dettweiler, exercise and rest, and, however improbably, reconciled them.

And it also addressed another perennial dilemma of medical care: how does the doctor, authority and expert, cope with the bottomless uncertainties of mortal illness? At the turn of the twentieth century, faced with the lessening but still essentially unmanageable ravages of consumption, physicians may have understood in accurate detail the cause and the progress of the disease; but their understanding as to how and why it worked was far less specific than their understanding of its etiology. To maintain their authority as practitioners, as healers, rather than as mere theoreticians or pathologists, they needed to be as specific and methodical in their cures as they were in their diagnoses, and this proved elusive. The rest-cure ritual filled the gap; if the patient wanted a regimen to follow, most doctors were, in the absence of any empirically tested therapy, only too happy to provide them with it. The doctors knew perfectly well how incomplete their knowledge was, how notoriously hard it was to predict the outcome of a given case of tuberculosis. Apparently vigorous patients with minor cases might rapidly worsen and die; weaklings in a state of advanced debilitation might improve. It was hard to explain the exact mechanism of cures when they occurred, and equally hard to explain relapses. So the physician always hungered after more method than science had so far afforded him: it had uncovered so much that it came, perhaps, to seem that method itself, in any form, was salubrious.

The sanatorium was born at the beginning of a new age of scientific medicine; yet the disease it treated was not to succumb to science for nearly a century. As a result, though founded on science, the sanatorium looked for practical measures to tradition, to general ideas about what constituted health rather than specific therapies. It was modern, to a degree technical and bureaucratic, but it was also a folk institution, rooted in cultural beliefs about health not yet replaced by scientific professionalism. Hospitals rode the crest of technological progress into the twentieth century; they have survived and come to dominate the field of institutional health care. But the sanatorium kept its links with folk tradition; its mania for method, though pervasive, was rooted in common sense and popular belief rather than specialized knowledge. And if it was fated to disappear, rendered superfluous by antibiotics, it offered its patients a hominess, a relative informality, a version of normalcy alien to the modern hospital, but one that the modern hospital might do well to rediscover. Nowhere is this plainer than in the responses the patients gave to their stays within the walls of sanatoriums.

4

"Our Serene Life":
Rituals of the Cure

... Swing Into Action! . . . San Dust . . . Along the
Magic Way . . . Prayer . . . Chimes O' McGregor . . .
Our Serene Life . . .

—DEPARTMENTS IN
The Optimist,
THE MOUNT MCGREGOR SANATORIUM
MAGAZINE (1938–39)

NOTICE TO ACCEPTED CANDIDATES
FOR OTISVILLE SANATORIUM
READ THIS NOTICE CAREFULLY

You have been accepted as a suitable case for treatment
at Otisville Sanatorium. Your name has been placed on a
waiting list. When a vacancy occurs you will be notified to
present yourself at the Admission Bureau, 426 First Avenue, Borough of Manhattan, for Admission.

If under the influence of liquor or smelling of the same
you will be rejected. You must not take liquor with you.

All patients who have been accepted must supply
themselves with a complete outfit of articles described in
this circular.

These outfits should be packed in a suit case or bundle.
They will be inspected at the Admission Bureau on the
day you start for Otisville Sanatorium. *Do not bring a
trunk.*

So, in 1914, came the good news of acceptance for treatment
at New York City's municipal sanatorium in the Catskills. Otis-

ville admitted only charity patients and ran itself according to the brisk principles laid down by the city's leading antituberculosis crusader, Dr. Hermann M. Biggs. But in its emphasis on discipline, in its call to a simple and healthfully controlled existence, it was characteristic: the patient's new life called to him in a voice of thunder. Sanatorium routine was a decisive break with the past, a carefully marked and exclamatory farewell to the normal.

In the Middle Ages, unfortunates diagnosed as having leprosy were forced to live apart, in an exile colony outside the city walls, the banishment inaugurated by a mock funeral rite. The stricken leper, clad in burial weeds, was forced to view his own symbolic burial, then driven from the city to live among the marked and the shunned. Underneath the apparent cruelty of this there was perhaps a hidden if unsparing kindness. For the sake of the common good there had to be a wrenching break, and it was perhaps in the long run more charitable to recognize it openly and commemorate it ceremonially, bringing the trauma into the light rather than suppressing it.

Otisville's announcement, less darkly, served the same purpose—the break it called for was just as decisive, the life the patient was about to embark on just as Spartan. Men were told to bring with them a single suit of clothes, a cap, three shirts, three suits of underwear, three pairs of socks, two suits of overalls and pajamas; one pair each of shoes and rubbers. A few layers of outerwear were added if the cure commenced in winter; the list of necessaries for women was a little, but not much, longer. (It required, for reasons not specified, much more underwear.)

When the new patient arrived at the hospital encampment, he found an attractive mountain setting but rudimentary accommodations. The universal sanatorium plan had been followed, but pared down to eliminate architectural flourishes of the sort that had made the Adirondack Cottage Sanatorium a showplace. Otisville offered the Outdoor Life in its pure form, but without the distracting amenities. The men's dormitories had no plumbing, for reasons explained by the medical director:

> The living and dressing rooms were heated but experience soon showed that during cold weather the patients, unless watched, frequently lounged in the warm dressing room, and so to insure continuous life in the open, orders were issued that the windows and doors of the living and dressing rooms should be kept wide open throughout the day from 9 A.M. to 5 P.M. With the intensely cold weather prevailing at Otisville in winter, this regulation resulted in the freezing of the pipes, and this led to the abandonment of plumbing fixtures in most of the subsequent buildings.

Otisville's routine was typical, a version of the daily schedule observed at dozens of sanatoriums between 1900 and 1925. The first week the patient spent largely in bed, allowing his condition to be assessed and enabling the hospital to establish a base line for vital statistics like weight and temperature. Thereafter the patient's activity gradually increased (more quickly at Otisville than was typical, since the philosophy here was that indigent patients should be put to work as soon as possible during the cure, lest habits of idleness set in). For most of the stay, a patient divided his day between periods of absolute rest and of carefully graded activity, spending as much time as possible in the open air.

Patients rose to a bell at 6:30 each morning. Except for the few confined absolutely to bed, they ate in communal dining halls (segregated by sex) in two shifts between 7:00 and 7:30 or 8:00 and 8:30. Directly after breakfast came a daily ritual, the exchange of sputum cups: yesterday's handed in for destruction, clean ones issued. Between 9:00 and 10:00 the medical staff made its rounds; from 10:00 to 12:00 the patients rested or performed such work as the hospital thought advisable. The main meal took place shortly after noon; more work or rest followed between 2:00 and 5:00; supper came between 5:00 and 6:00. Thereafter the patients rested or entertained themselves until 9:15, when a warning bell sounded. At 9:30 there was a second bell and all the lights went off.

A regimented life, not accidentally reminiscent of monastic routine, even to the segregation of the sexes, and accompanied by rules no less comprehensive for being simple and few in number: at Otisville there were only ten, but they covered every eventuality. Patients were required to pay strict attention to the sanitary disposal of their sputum; to remain in the open air at all times except from supper to bedtime; to wash their hands before and brush their teeth after meals. The rules were seen not simply as conveniences for the institution or laws governing the social lives of the patients but as an essential part of the cure. "Your chances of getting well depend largely upon the observance of these rules. It is, therefore, to your interest to obey them and to see that they are followed by the other patients. The individual who breaks these rules is your enemy, and should be reported at once."

Beginning the cure was, on the one hand, an occasion of good luck, anticipated and much looked forward to: the waiting periods, sometimes protracted, required by the press of applicants on the better-known sanatoriums, made the summons a source of joy when it came. But on the other it was like beginning a sentence to penal servitude. It meant confinement for an indefinite period and submission to rigid regulation. Complexity and unpredictability shrank within the ambit of the hospital routine, and in theory, at least, the only possible source of drama or surprise was the behavior of your untrustworthy lungs. You were, in the typical sanatorium, surrounded by open space, but you viewed it, if you followed Lawrason Brown's bundling-up instructions, from an envelope as secure (and as confining) as a cocoon or an infant's swaddling clothes. If the cure proceeded according to plan, you gained weight, but lost your independence, regressing, in your relation to the hospital staff, to moral childhood. Your sense of time changed—hours, days, and even weeks lost their shape, to be replaced by a framework of months and years.

Patients, unsurprisingly, reacted very differently to the

shock. The "sick role," as Talcott Parsons once defined it, offers the relief of exemption from normal social obligations, but it also designates you as one in need of help and hence places you in subjection to the will of your healers. Some newly institutionalized "lungers" rebelled, but that, granted the rigidities of the sanatorium regimen and the fact that consumption was often a disease of few incapacitating symptoms, was to be expected. More surprising is the majority of surviving ex-patients who report that they followed the discipline equably and remember their stays affectionately. Most of them appear to have accepted the teaching of relentless optimism and good spirits and enjoyed, though ambiguously, the return to implied childhood and adolescence. Living by rules, advancing cautiously and under the discerning doctor's paternal eye, from complete dependence to gradually increasing activity, was like growing up from infancy again. This proved in most cases oddly exhilarating, perhaps simply because it promised a new beginning to people stricken, often in their prime, with a disease that threatened the catastrophic end of everything.

In 1954, on the fiftieth anniversary of the founding of Ray Brook, the New York State public sanatorium near Saranac Lake, Henry Levy, an ex-patient, recalled his arrival in 1931. His description is a folk version of the sanatorium arrival immortalized at the beginning of *The Magic Mountain,* but with no overlay of literary self-consciousness:

> My first glimpse of the small cubicle of a station buried in heavily falling snow, stuck seemingly in a cold wilderness, was far from comforting.
> Who hasn't conjectured as to what one may expect to find? All you know, you've got a dreaded disease and you're going to a hospital or San. The name commonly used then was consumption, which left a lump in your throat at the mere sound of it.

But, in memory, the dread and doom give way to immediate reassurance, warmth, comfort, cure. Reminiscences by typical alumni of the sanatoriums skip over the setbacks, the inter-ludes of depression or despair, and willingly adopt the opti-mism all sanatoriums promulgated as official policy:

> The ride from the station up the hill to the main entrance was over before I knew it. I was ushered in and instead of cold forboding [*sic*] walls, was amazed at the warm reception by a doctor. The interior itself looked more like a sumptious [*sic*] spacious comfortable lodge than a hospi-tal as there was nothing to indicate the latter, even to the pungent smell of drugs or ether. The fountain in the Cen-ter Building playing silent thin streams of water over a bronze boy holding an umbrella, into a wide circular base where goldfish swam about lazily, fascinated me. This in-deed was the farthest I ever saw of a hospital. The only indication that I was in one was when the nurse came over to escort me to my quarters in Pryor Wing. After nine months I was on my way home, "fit as a fiddle."

Thanks to Thomas Mann, the sanatorium lingers in public consciousness as an automatic metaphor, poised midway be-tween the nineteenth and twentieth centuries, balanced deli-cately along the line between life and death, a place for elabo-rate philosophizing. But the American sanatorium, though, of course, ultimate dramas lay behind it, was a folk institution. Great issues simplified themselves into bright colors; plain peo-ple felt at home there, resolutely shaking off the terrors and determined that the exile should not be an escape from the normal, but, as far as possible, a reassertion of it.

Naturally, few average patients wrote at length about their experiences; the ones who did were exceptions. But a few left memoirs that seem to reflect the experience of the typical sanatorium patient, and among these perhaps the most inter-esting, because the least literary, was Isabel Smith's.

Struck with tuberculosis in 1928 while a student nurse in New York, she moved to Saranac Lake and, awaiting admission to the Adirondack Cottage Sanatorium, began treatment at one of the town's privately run boardinghouses for the tuber-cular. Her doctor, Francis B. Trudeau, was Edward Livingston's son and successor. She remained for three years under his care at her cure cottage until, in 1931, she moved to the Trudeau Sanatorium, where, apart from a few short breaks, she was to spend the next eighteen years. A *Life* magazine spread in 1937, photographed by Alfred Eisenstaedt, included two memorable pictures of her, one staring out at the mountain landscape, the other lying transparently asleep. This earned her a fleeting fame, some fan letters (picturesque invalids had not lost their allure in the 1930s), even a transient suitor. Eventually, in a pattern classic among the consumptive, she fell in love with and married a fellow patient, Courtney Malmstrom. In 1949 she was, thanks to successful therapy with the new generation of antibiotics, able to leave the hospital; like many of its alumni, the Malmstroms remained indissolubly attached to the town and its way of life.

Smith responded to her doctors and to the cure itself exactly as the manuals said she should: docilely. She spent most of her three years in the cure cottage on St. Bernard Street flat on her back, but recalled the ordeal fondly, blotting out the darker recollections with warm memories, not the less touching because they're synthetic. "A smiling buxom woman, with lovely dark eyes, opened the door and as I caught sight of her white uniform I felt reassured," she writes of her arrival at the boardinghouse. The waiting period for admission to the sanatorium, agonizing and anxiety-ridden for most patients, was for her a pleasant three-year interlude; she grew attached to the cottage, its proprietor, its occupants, and the solicitous visits from Francis Trudeau. The announcement that she was finally to enter the sanatorium came as an unpleasant shock. A new room, roommate, a new nurse, a new doctor—all were threatening, small changes made gigantic by the preceding inactivity.

> The room, with its pale painted walls was filled with sunshine, but it looked lonely and bare. To make things worse, as the great collection of belongings, which I had somehow accumulated, was unpacked, I was informed that many of the familiar objects which had made my former dwelling into a home must now be stored out of

sight. I flounced pouting into bed and lay there, staring at the ceiling, hating every crack. My dinner tray arrived. I took one look and refused to eat.

Smith's book, *Wish I Might,* is an extended version of the short articles that filled the *Journal of the Outdoor Life,* the national sanatorium magazine, and the mimeographed institutional journals put out at most hospitals. All of them affect a folkish immediacy, everyman's idea of the literary—Henry Levy's memory of the fountain in Center Building at Ray Brook, Isabel Smith's self-consciously lively prose: "hating every crack." Are they recalling real emotions, or the therapeutic fabrication of optimism as required by the cure? Is Smith's ironic memory of her petulance upon admission to the Trudeau Sanatorium genuinely that, or the good patient's determination to see her own rebellion from the hospital's point of view?

Smith had not, except for her brief spell as a student nurse, done anything or been anywhere. From the moment she came down with it, she applied herself to tuberculosis as a career, sunniness as her work. The sanatoriums insisted that the cure was a kind of business, an activity, a profession for which real skills could be acquired and practiced, and Smith's memoirs are a practical reflection of that belief. What she writes is what, in the sanatorium's view, she ought to write—a tale of optimism and cooperativeness. The vapors and the blues are allowed in, but only to be mocked away. Whatever temptations may have existed toward real despair are left in the spaces the book doesn't fill: Smith quickly counteracts her initial sullen resentment at the confinements of her new room. The nurse wheels her out onto the sleeping porch, and

> as my bed neared the windows, suddenly I beheld the mountains! I was actually *seeing* them at last! The impact of their size and color under the bright October sun knocked the chip right off my shoulder. I cried out in surprise and delight. Stalwart and reassuring they stood awaiting me, the darkness of evergreen mottling their

contours, their sides splashed with patches of crimson, russet and gold. . . . It seemed almost too good to be true that I could lie here and look at all this wonder and beauty just as long as I liked.

Surrounded by scenery that suggests wholeness and health, Smith is suggesting, you absorbed it imaginatively, eventually vanquishing the reality of the disease. A failure to adopt the ambient optimism was a failure in the cure, and the patient who chose to dwell on grim realities was not just imaginatively deficient but medically remiss. As with a monastic regimen, the rules aimed as much at a spiritual triumph as at a regulation of the physical disposition of life.

A poem by a South Carolina patient struck this theme:

> If you want to cure in the kind of a San
>   Like the kind of a San you like
> You needn't pack your clothes in a grip
>   And start on a long, long hike.
> You'll only find what you left behind,
>   For there is nothing that is really new.
> It's a knock at yourself when you knock the San,
>   It isn't the San, it's you.

The sanatoriums were health institutions, steeped in the scientific bias the medical profession affected in the late nineteenth and early twentieth centuries. But they aspired beyond that to enroll patients in a movement, to stimulate their imaginations, to embark on a metaphorical crusade. Doggerel verse and giddy inspiration pieces poured forth from the invalids and were an important appurtenance of the cure. All sanatoriums published magazines; contributions were actively sought from patients and were always accepted as long as they seemed spontaneous, fostered camaraderie, toed the optimistic line, and avoided the appearance of professionalism. Isabel Smith's book is simply the most extended example of a widespread genre.

Isabel Smith suffered twenty years of nearly incessant discouragement and boredom, punctuated by catastrophic setbacks (after emerging from the strict confinement of the Tru-

deau infirmary to the relative freedom of a rest cottage, she
suffered a relapse and was sent back to bed rest once again).
Turning her experiences into a journal of nearly unbroken
optimism, a *Candide* without irony, was no small trick. A surgeon removes eleven of her ribs; World War II breaks out; her
mother dies; the bombs fall on Hiroshima and Nagasaki. But
her reaction, in each case heartily approved of by the sanatorium staff, is to put the tragedy, her own and the world's,
behind her and embark, within her capacities, on an improving project. The nuclear attack on Japan stimulated her to
embark on a study of nuclear energy. Not, of course, a taxing
or rigorous one—her prescribed text was George Gamov's *Mr.
Tompkins in Wonderland.* Bedridden and thus deprived even
of her mountain view, she enjoys a terrarium: "From that time
on for months I walked in fancy through the paths of my
terrarium. I rested beneath a seedling tree and skipped over
the stones in the brook. Sometimes my patch of woodland was
dry, but more often it sparkled with myriad drops as though
a shower had just passed. Even when I closed my eyes its
greenness remained with me—its pebbles shining white, its
partridge berries sharply red." The terrarium's scaled-down,
walled-off nature echoed the whole sanatorium experience,
every vista panoramic but walled off from the observer, distant, always seen as if in miniature.

This ironclad determination to tear contentment through
the iron gates of despair is a thrust against illness; but yet it's
also a symptom of it. The very energy of the refusal to acknowledge despair testifies to its nearness and power. Early in her
life at Saranac, Smith decided to keep a notebook devoted to
dark thoughts not allowed into public currency by the sanatorium. "It would be my Trouble Book. In it I would set down
all my tumultuous, chaotic thoughts just as they came,
stripped, as far as I could achieve it, of all illusion and pretense.
I could afford to be honest for no one was *ever* to see what
would be written there." Invisibility was the essence of the
Trouble Book. Unspoken, unseen, its contents have no power
to corrupt the metaphor of wholeness being painstakingly cul-
tivated in the sanatorium ("health" is etymologically identical

with "wholeness"). "Writing in my Trouble Book provided me with a means for taking action of a sort, even when it did not amount to more than pushing a pen. And when I closed its pages I always felt relieved and released, as if whatever I had confided to it was now no longer *here,* but *there.*" To write something down, in other words, is to confine it safely to unreality. Consumption had, and still has, the reputation of a literary disease, a condition that lends itself to metaphor. But sanatorium residents were encouraged to think of it as the very reverse: the language in which it was to be recorded was inflexibly light, inconsequential, and disposable. If darker-than-allowed emotions reared themselves, they might be deprived of their power by writing them down, but the danger to public morale could be eliminated by keeping them secret.

Clara N. Bates, an Oklahoma patient who had completed a three-year-long cure, wrote a short story, "It Can Be Done," about the laudable determination of a fictional but plainly autobiographical Alicia May.

> When the porch was ready for its new occupant Alicia smiled a gay little smile, but her eyes were hard and bright.
> "I'll never let anyone know, I'll bear all this alone. Life, you have cheated me," she said. "But the game isn't finished. I can cheat, too. I am going to pretend to be glad!"
> So, to Alicia, the days resolved themselves into an odd little secret game. With merry whimsicality she played against the silent opponent. The slow hours of lassitude, the heavy hours of pain, the black depression that was hardest of all to bear, she lost, so she said, to the enemy, the great gray shadow who played against her.

Alicia May's optimism is a conscious artifice, a defiant rejection of unacceptable truth, grounded in the faith that the specious, dutifully maintained, can become real.

> Her friends found she turned a willing ear to [the] hopeful . . . was oddly . . . inattentive to morbid stories, faultfinding, gossip, and detailed accounts of illnesses. . . . And so

108

Alicia played her game and won. Bless you, yes, of course she won!

Intriguingly, in European accounts of sanatorium life, grim realism replaces the Kiwanis-like optimism of the American accounts. A 1942 memoir by Alan Dick, a British veteran of World War I, illustrates this. In transit to his sanatorium, Dick amuses himself by sticking his tongue out at pedestrians through the one-way window of his ambulance. Once installed there, he follows a routine essentially the same as the American one, but he, his fellow patients, and his doctors preserve a skeptical distance from it, as emerges when he contemplates the sanatorium's famous view, of rolling farmland.

> Beside me was the farmer's son whom I had noticed on my first visit to the dining room. As my eyes travelled over the unspoiled valley stretching away to the smoke-grey escarpment I turned to him and exclaimed: "Isn't that grand country!" After I had spoken he surveyed the scene with mild appraisement, pursed his lips shrewdly and replied: "Ten bob an acre stuff."

Dick's physician dismisses him from the sanatorium with the same advice in substance as every discharged patient received: the discipline of the cure was to be carried over into life. But the English doctor's valedictory is laconic and understated:

> You went into hospital a sick man. You had a dangerous disease which would have got you if it had gone on. The doctors gave you treatment which got you out of bed, put you on your feet, and made you fit to work. You owe it to them not to undo the good work they have done you by larking about and being silly.

The evenness of both the patient's and the physician's attitude is uncharacteristic of the American experience, in which the ideology of the cure looms over its clinical method. After all, American awareness of tuberculosis had been created by a publicity campaign, founded on hyperbole, and hyperbole remained with it.

But occasionally the dark underside of the cure found expression as well, less frequently but more forcefully, and with a characteristic intensity, going as far beyond the European matter-of-factness in unflinching grimness as Isabel Smith fell short of it. Perhaps the best, certainly the most striking and least conventional of all the American sanatorium memoirs was Betty MacDonald's *The Plague and I* (1948). Like Isabel Smith's, MacDonald's sanatorium stay took place in the 1930s; but hers was shorter (she left, her disease arrested, within a year), and she was altogether a more mordant observer than Smith, more willing to face the contradictions underlying the ideology of the cure. *The Plague and I* takes as its raw material the same images that the sanatoriums purveyed in their propaganda, that patients and physicians included in their recollections. But MacDonald infuses those images with an awareness of the horrors beneath, stretching and distorting them until, as if against their own will, they reveal the abysses Smith dutifully confined to the secret pages of her Trouble Book.

MacDonald was a patient at Firland, the King County sanatorium north of Seattle proper (in the book it's called the Pines). Her recollection of her first glimpse of its buildings and grounds captures the Elysian qualities the architects sought in their designs but also includes a tenebrous countertheme:

> We entered the Pines by a long, poplar-lined drive. On either side were great vine-covered Tudor buildings, rolling lawns, greenhouses and magnificent gardens. It might have been any small endowed college except that there were no laughing groups strolling under the trees. In fact the only sign of life anywhere at all was a single nurse who flitted between two buildings like a white paper in the wind.

Catatonia enthralls the place, undispelled by the hominess of its design. Symbols of normalcy are turned hallucinatory by disuse:

> The waiting room had large casement windows, a lovely view of the gardens, overstuffed furniture, a virginal fire-

place with its firebricks washed and waxed clear up into the chimney, and no magazines, no ashtrays. We put down the suitcases, chose places, sat down and were immediately engulfed in silence. The kind of all-embracing silence that makes the sound of a purse clasp sound like a pistol shot, the scratch of a match like the rasp of a hacksaw blade. Mary said at last, in a strained unnatural voice, "Napoleon Bonaparte had tuberculosis but I don't suppose you care. I certainly don't." The silence settled down again like wet newspapers. Finally Madge, who was young and healthy but a terrific hypochondriac, said in her deep, slow voice, "God this is a depressing place! It would cheer me up just to hear somebody choking to death. Sydney, do you think I've got t.b.?" Mother said, "Madge, you know that if this were an orthopedic hospital the pain would be in your leg." Madge laughed and dropped all the books again. No one came. Nothing happened. Just the silence.

The conventional and approved response to the hospital routine was that it was well paced, so accurate a miniature of life outside the grounds that you could, once you accommodated yourself to the reduced scale, imagine yourself living normally, not immobilized but ceaselessly active. In *Saints Rest*, Sadie Fuller Seagrave's 1918 reminiscence of sanatorium life thinly disguised as a novel, Rose, the patient heroine, writes her fiancé shortly after her arrival:

Really one doesn't have as much time as might be expected. You see in the morning after breakfast we must make our beds, do our share of cleaning up the cottage, then take our exercise, then undress and go to bed and be absolutely quiet for half an hour. Then we must record our temperature and pulse. Between then and dinner time I have a little extra time because so far I have not taken much exercise. . . . After dinner we have to undress again and go to bed until 3 or 4 o'clock. I haven't [had] any afternoon exercise yet, so I have a little time before supper, which is generally the time I write letters. After supper it is to bed again for an hour. Then we can be up until nine but the lights must go out at nine, sharp. O, talk about a well-regulated life! A 65 dollar Swiss watch can't begin to compete with us.

Compare Betty MacDonald's harrowing sense of time during the rest hours at the Pines; instead of placidity, contentment, even pride, they breed rage:

> I had to remind myself to be grateful because my instinct was to be resentful. Resentful of the rules, resentful of the nurses who enforced the rules. What was the matter with me? Was that what the Medical Director had meant when he said the cure would be hard for me, or were all tuberculosis patients the same way? I would ask. . . . When the rest hours were over. I looked at my watch. It was one-seven. I looked back at the ceiling and tried to relax my fingers but my heart was pounding and I felt like a sky-rocket about to explode into a million jagged stars. I turned my pillow over and took another drink of the tepid water. . . . I reached out and got my damp cold washcloth and put it over my eyes. That was better. I thought, "That is my big toe. It is heavy." . . . I took the washcloth off and turned over so I could see the poplar tree again. While I watched, one small leaf let go and dropped limply through the misty air. Compared to the hospital it seemed like an act of hysterical activity.

To such overpowering ennui the Pines responds with maxims: each meal arrives together with a slip of paper bearing a beautiful thought. "IF YOU HAVE NOTHING TO DO, DON'T DO IT HERE." "IF YOU THINK RIGHT, YOU WILL ACT RIGHT."

The insistence on a stiff upper lip was, from the hospital's point of view, understandable and necessary, since one slip in your determination might release a pent-up torrent of destructive despair. So one patient, a Miss Emma S. Theiss, provoked a small controversy among the readers of the *Journal of the Outdoor Life* when she wrote to the magazine, wondering if other lungers shared her annoyance at the self-consciousness of the official optimism. Over the course of several months, various patients responded, the overwhelming majority strongly in favor of the official optimism, and surprisingly aware of the degree to which it was a falsehood, though a salutary one:

> Are you really in earnest when you say that you are tired of always looking for the sun, and the cloud's silver lining? I have been looking for the sun for years, and always hope to continue to do so.
>
> Two years ago I was called a hopeless case. My respiration was 48, and my average temperature 104°. But I always believe that where there's life there's hope. And by [a] continuous Pollyanna diet plus make-believe I am going to be the victor. Actual thought on the hopelessness of my case would have overwhelmed me. Each time I read an account of a patient being cured I am renewed with fresh strength and courage. I know that I can do what others have done. . . . So, I say, thank God for the Pollyannas and the Make-Believes. Thank Him for the JOURNAL OF THE OUTDOOR LIFE, which encourages patients to win the battle.

Patients willing to subscribe so readily to such an ideology were quick to accept personal authority as well, and in the familial world of the sanatorium the doctor filled the role of the stern but loving father. Where the conditions warranted it, he could turn more than parental, and become Mosaic. When Isabel Smith fell in love with and decided to marry Courtney Malmstrom, she turned first to Francis B. Trudeau, and the reaction she records is comically parental, a blend of kind and thunderous avuncularity:

> "I'm going to be married!" I cried, catching his hand in mine.
>
> There was silence. I looked up with a sinking heart. Why wasn't he whooping with delight? Instead he looked pale and there was alarm written in his face.
>
> "When?" he barked.

Only after many X rays and much delay is he persuaded: " 'All right, Izzy, dear,' he said." And finally the ceremony, in "Trudeau's lovely little chapel among all our friends, with flowers, organ music, and best of all, my wonderful, loyal doctor to give me away!" Only with difficulty can you get more Oedipal than to marry in a chapel named after your parent; but Smith was not bothered by the symbolism.

The doctor's authority could, of course, have its dark as well as its light side; Sadie Fuller Seagrave rendered the ambiguity by dividing her doctor in two. The brooding, authoritarian Dr. Leeds, arbitrary and tyrannical ("I always take the word of my nurses in preference to that of my patients."), is replaced midway through the book by the stern but benevolent Dr. Murdock:

> He doesn't set himself up like an autocrat, and he realizes that it is much easier to follow instructions when you see a reason for them, and he is always ready to explain, and the more ignorant the person, the more patient and forebearing he is.

If the doctor's strength and authority compensated for the patient's vulnerability, however, it also underscored it, reminding him of his frailty and the nearness of death. In *The Plague and I*, death—a taboo subject in official sanatorium literature—does appear, and in the most frightening possible guise, as a nightmare image of the white-coated doctor. Both patrol the wards, the healer during the day, the destroyer at night. MacDonald's acerbic Japanese wardmate, Kimi, first voices this idea:

> To me Death is a lecherous, sly, deranged old man. His beard is sparse and stained. His eyes are coarse-lidded, red rimmed, furtive and evil. His loose red lips are slimy and drooling. He pants with anticipation. . . . He shuffles up and down the corridor at night, his malodorous, black robe dragging behind him. . . . Each time Margaretta or any other very sick patient passes our door I fancy I see Death's evil face peering around the corner. I . . . can see him hovering like a great bat over the emergency ward, the light room, the private room. I can hear him shuffling up and down the corridor at night.

MacDonald, intrigued by this ghoulish image, finds it haunting her, a nocturnal counterpoint to the sanatorium's daytime diet of rest, wholesome pastimes, and Beautiful Thoughts. It provokes exactly the kind of thought in which inspirational patients were not supposed to indulge.

I awoke in the cold, early night to the dark stillness of the ward. I always hated the Pines at night. It was so much a hospital where anything might happen, anyone might die. . . . The Barking Dog began to cough, her coughs bursting from her like balls from a Roman candle. She coughed twenty-two times, then drank water and put the glass back on the stand with a clink. The woman across from her coughed, drank water, and coughed again. . . . Finally everyone seemed to be awake and there were coughs up and down the halls like a relay race. A grim terrible race with Death holding the stakes. I thought of Eileen cold and alone with sandbags on her chest. Sylvia had said that hemorrhages were very frightening. That the blood was bright red and foamy.

Someone was tapping on her stand. It was the way to summon a nurse but never used, especially at night, except in an emergency. The tapping went on, clink, clink, clink, clink. It seemed to come from down the hall where the private rooms were. Eleanor said in a whisper, "Something's happened. I hear a doctor." . . .

Morning came at last, dark and wild with wind and rain lashing and clawing at the windows. The ward was oppressively quiet. The day staff came on duty, cheerful and brisk, bringing breakfast. I gulped down two cups of warm comforting coffee but I couldn't shake the horror of the night before. I . . . thought I detected an ominous undercurrent. There was a furtiveness to the whispering. In the bathroom I learned, from one of the older patients, that a girl in emergency had died during the night. I had never seen the girl, didn't even know her name but it was my first death. My slowly built up confidence and assurance of recovery were kicked from under me, I shivered uncontrollably. . . .

Jarring notes like MacDonald's are rare in the literature of the antituberculosis movement; from the 1880s through its decline in the 1950s, its idiom is surprisingly consistent. Deaths, grotesque and disturbing incidents, oddly fail to contaminate the memory. One Saranac Lake alumnus, interviewed for a local television documentary, recalled the town's lively social atmosphere, the youth of the patients. He then talked of a female patient, who, despairing of a cure, lay down on the railroad tracks near the station, waiting there patiently as the train approached from several miles down the track. Why, he wonders, would she ever want to kill herself? Another woman, who worked in the 1940s as a student nurse at the Mount Morris sanatorium near Rochester, recalled swimming in the sanatorium's man-made lake, romances between patients and staff, good food, and attractive grounds. Yet her most specific memory was of a child visiting a parent, forced to stand on the grass outside the hospital, talking to the patient through the screens on the sleeping porch. Optimism didn't succeed in, and probably didn't aim at, eradicating the memory of suffering; it simply neutralized it, rendering it harmless without obliterating it.

Did it work, this iatrogenic repression of dark thoughts? Did resolute Panglossianism arm the body against the disease? Statistics are inconclusive but on balance not reassuring. Consistently, from the beginning of the sanatorium movement through the 1940s, nearly 25 percent of all patients died while in the hospital, and 50 percent of all released patients succumbed within five years of discharge. Some institutions prided themselves on records better than this average, but these were often the ones that limited patients, as far as possible, to those with incipient tuberculosis, and left the moribund to state and county hospitals. The persistence of such high mortality rates, despite declines in the number of new cases and alleged improvements in the cure, suggests that MacDonald's skepticism was well founded if bad for morale.

For those who survived the whole of a sanatorium stay and mended sufficiently to merit a discharge, the time they looked back on was a journal of progress, a symbolic childhood, beginning with infancy, passing a mock adolescence, ending, when

116

they left the sanatorium, with a reemergence into independent adulthood. As the notice to new patients from Otisville suggested, the complete break with the past one made upon admission prepared one to start afresh. And the first stage of the cure, as short as a week or two in some hospitals, but lasting for months in others, was a period of complete bed rest. It was a state approaching babyhood—you ate in bed, were bathed and excreted in bed, and were wheeled inside or out as was thought appropriate.

Then, immediately, childhood began. The Trudeau routine was universal—as one patient remembered it, a nurse called on him

> with a rule book, which I was supposed to read and sign. It had my number on it—8027. I felt worse than ever. Like a prison. And the book was full of rules, lots of rules. Everyone must be out of doors, except those working in offices or workshops, between 9 and 12:30 and between 2 and 5. Everyone was expected to go to bed in the afternoon. No one could leave the grounds to go to town unless he had at least half an hour exercise. No one was allowed off the grounds after 7:30 without a pass and no more than six passes could be given each month. Visiting between the sexes was allowed only on porches of cottages between 3:30 and 5 o'clock in the afternoon.

There were two rationales for this pseudogestation. One was the value of absolute rest as the most reliable way to stabilize the tubercular process in the lungs; another was the need for an objective evaluation of the patient's underlying condition, freed as far as possible from environmental stresses. But for the patient, it was a shock. You were not allowed to glide effortlessly into the discipline of the cure, but were forced to adjust all at once; and doing so was, for many patients, a hard-won victory.

Marian Spitzer, a screenwriter and journalist, fell ill in 1937; although she followed the cure at home under the supervision of a hired doctor and nurse, her regimen was essentially the same as would be followed at a sanatorium. For her the shock

117

of moving directly from an active life to complete bed rest had its own logic; the drama of the change made it easier to adjust to the thought of living with illness: "From a purely practical point of view it seems to me a sense of humor is less useful to a TB victim than a sense of drama. There are certain situations you simply can't laugh your way out of."

Bed rest set the stage for this struggle. As virtually all patients recall it, even Isabel Smith, the confinement and ennui of the first few weeks became a battle between the patient and the hospital, which, if successful, the patient lost, allowing him to make a definitive break with the past and embark on life in a new dimension. The patient would not internalize the philosophy of the cure unless he first vented his resistance to it. "Pretty nearly all TB patients regard their doctors as enemies at first," Spitzer says, "and most of the doctors know it." Her doctor formulates the situation for her, and his lecture shares themes common in patients' memories of the talking-to the doctor supplies in response to their early rebelliousness: "You *have* an enemy, . . . a very vicious enemy inside you, working night and day to destroy you. And you have a choice. You can join that enemy and work against me—and yourself. Or you can join me and work against the enemy."

The successful patient, after tremors of insurrection, won the battle over his own intransigence, and allied himself with the hospital and the doctor against the illness. The triumph had something of the absoluteness of religious conversion, and the convert turned his back on the old life as he embraced the new one:

> The language of the sanatorium is unique and not always intelligible to the uninitiated. The newcomer is bewildered by it; if someone has "chucked a ruby" he does not understand it; and to be told to "hit the hay and stay put" he finds to be the equivalent of several paragraphs of detailed instruction said in more elegant language. But he learns it, he uses it, he writes it to his friends and family, for it is one of the interesting things learned in sanatorium life.

In his account of the sanatorium routine, Dr. John Potts distinguished among patient types. The indifferent, the overeager, and the rebellious were all, in his view, doomed to relapse and ultimate death. Success is most often reserved to representatives of what he calls the "Soldier Type": "They say to their medical attendant: 'I am like a soldier; I want definite orders given me, and then I will carry them out.'" More successful still was the "Reading Type," who, like the Good Soldier, follows orders, but with a salt of intelligence. His acquiescence in the regime is more valuable because it is well informed. "These patients . . . have good self-control, a detailed knowledge of what to do and what not to do in the daily routine, and they use good judgment, not because one doctor has told them what to do, but because they have found that other doctors through the printed page have given the same instruction."

This hard-won, conscious passivity was the real psychological goal of the cure; achieving it was a struggle good patients are proud to have won. Marian Spitzer's early insurrectionist impulses finally erupted in a few infantile defiances—secretly brushing her own hair and sneaking a few phone calls. When she finally collapsed in the middle of an attempt to pick up the phone, her physician told her he'd known all along she was cheating, because her pulse and temperature records divulged it. "A chart is rather like a lie detector, you know."

The interlocked rule-following and rebellion were so suggestive of adolescence that patients and doctors both remarked it. Romances, for instance, though discouraged as an interruption of the cure and interfered with as far as possible by rules, nonetheless flourished. At Trudeau, the practice became a sort of undergraduate ritual with its own argot: your lover was a "cousin," the affair itself was called "cousining," and the favorite trysting place on the Trudeau grounds, a small rest pavilion, was the "Cousinola."

If you adjusted successfully to the early stages of the cure, and your temperature fell, your weight went up, the bacteria count in your sputum (called the Gaffky count, after the inventor of the test) went down, you were allowed more independence and more exercise and could begin to think of such diversions. At some sanatoriums, like Otisville, you were actually required to work as you got stronger, but at most you followed leisurely pursuits—cards, piano- and record-playing, parties, picnics. You could get a town permit and, at least in consumption-tolerant Saranac Lake, visit a restaurant or a movie theater. Every new patient at Trudeau was enrolled as a member of the Thursday Evening Club, which sponsored the hospital social activities, holiday parties, and special events, like the celebrations staged for discharged patients, called "Graduation Exercises." (A 1925 program included a mouth organ recital, a medley of Scotch airs, a presentation of X-ray plates, and a recitation contest, including "Symptoms," "My Fibrosis," "Da Fruita Stand," and "Lazy Moe.")

But at no matter what stage of the cure, everything in the sanatorium routine came to be invested with the aura of ritual, elaborating itself in details not strictly justified by clinical considerations. Lawrason Brown's elaborate instructions for wrapping oneself up in blankets on the cure porch is a case in point; so is the compulsive attention toward the details of diet. Charles T. Ryder and Gerald B. Webb put out in the 1920s a popular product called *Overcoming Tuberculosis: An Almanac of Recovery.* It consisted of a hortatory introduction followed by a series of charts, which, day by day, recorded a patient's weight and his morning and evening temperature. At the top and bottom of each weekly chart were helpful and bracing quotations from both literary and scientific sources. "It's the melancholy face gets stung by the bee" appears at the top of one chart; "The widespread ignorance of the harmfulness of exercise in the febrile stage of consumption is shocking" and "Ne'er-do-wells and failures in all walks of life are notorious advisers" at the bottom. Not all sanatoriums permitted patients to know their weight and temperature readings, on the theory that knowledge might be dispiriting, but others encouraged the habit of record keeping. It gave the patient something to do, implicated him in his own treatment, and fit in with the general compulsiveness of the routine. Marian Spitzer used *Overcoming Tuberculosis* during her confinement and reported that after suppressing an initial annoyance at its Panglossian advice, she found the process reassuring.

For the majority of the sanatorium inpatients, at least through the 1920s, the routine was the totality of the cure. It was, for the twentieth century, a remarkably untechnical form of therapy, not relying on machinery or drugs, invoking nature rather than the doctor's intervention. Though emphases differed, the very similarity of the regimen from hospital to hospital and state to state inspired solidarity: meals, the rituals of weekly weighing and temperature taking, the issuing and handing in of sputum cups, the alternation of rest hours with periods of limited but gradually increasing activity—all remained the hallmark of the sanatorium.

Yet even patients confined to their beds enjoyed some activity. By the early 1920s this had taken the form of occupational therapy, and it rapidly became a fixture of sanatorium life. Patients were encouraged, at times forced, to make things in bed, as a way of passing the time, releasing pent-up tension, at times even of supporting themselves. The *Journal of the Outdoor Life* ran a monthly column called "Let's Make Something"; some of the larger hospitals hired occupational-therapy instructors who trained patients in the manufacture of various peculiar products. Betty MacDonald christened these "toecovers"—decorative objects of self-evident uselessness. The message the sanatorium toecover conveyed was twofold: on the one hand it bespoke industry, but on the other it communicated alienation from everyday life. Isabel Smith evinced delight at the prospect occupational therapy opened before her: "tooling and putting together wallets, small purses and similar articles of leather, . . . knitting, crocheting and embroidering, . . . silver and copper ornaments, leather book ends, desk sets and numerous other things." Betty MacDonald's list is more trenchant:

a crocheted napkin ring, . . . embroidered book marks,
. . . embroidered coat hangers, hand-painted shoe-trees
(always painted with a special paint that never dries),
home-made three-legged footstools with the legs spaced
unevenly so the footstool always lies on one side, cross-
stitched pictures of lumpy brown houses with "The houfe
by the fide of the road" worked in Olde Englishe underneath, . . . crocheted paper knife handle covers complete
with tassel, [and] poorly executed dolls whose voluminous
skirts are supposed to cover telephones.

Such descriptions are not fanciful. Among the comparable
projects offered in the 1920s in the "Let's Make Something"
column in the *Journal of the Outdoor Life* were quilted
sachets, embroidered pajamas, shoe trees adorned with satin
ribbon, crocheted coat-hanger covers, and stuffed dogs ("Hello
folks! Meet Jabbey, Boloney and Beelzebub! Aren't they
sweet?"). The Adirondack Cottage Sanatorium published a
mail-order catalogue offering patient-made goods, largely
pseudo-Indian souvenirs; a number of patients kept themselves in spending money by selling their products to visitors
or to other patients.

Like everything else in the sanatorium, occupational therapy had a history; if the sanatorium represented a rejection of
the city, its crafts were a symbolic rejection of large-scale industry and were rooted ultimately in the pre-Raphaelite
movement. William Morris's crafts manufactures were a rebellious gesture against mass production, a reassertion of cottage
industry, a revaluing of the homemade above the manufactured. When this idea crossed the Atlantic, it lodged in a different sort of brain. Elbert Hubbard, a Harvard dropout and
tireless self-promoter, impressed by Morris on a trip to England, transported the idea back to the United States and
founded the Roycrofters, a complex of shops at East Aurora,
New York, near Buffalo. In Hubbard's rendering, Morris's cultivation of painstaking detail and careful training gave way to
durability, simplicity, and Yankee practicality. Where the pre-
Raphaelites turned out gossamer lyrics, neomedieval wallpa-

per, textiles, and neo-Arthurian romances, the Roycrofters published volumes of salty aphorisms in the pragmatic tradition of Poor Richard, and not dissimilar in tone from the *Journal of the Outdoor Life*. Crafts were vulgarized, no longer the province of the painstakingly trained artisan, but simple useful objects the common man could make—key cases, book covers, belts, and inkpots.

The Roycrofters helped spawn a fashion for folk crafts, on which sanatorium planners quickly seized; in their hands its latent paradoxes became manifest. On the one hand, it was just what it pretended to be—a way to occupy the patient without taxing him. But it also had a hidden dimension: it placed the patient clearly in a hierarchy, thanks to the starkness of the contrast between his "work" and the sanatorium staff's. Doctors and nurses commanded the routines of the cure, dispensed the medicines, ran the machinery. The patients made Rubber Flower Boutonnieres and Pine Cone Turkeys. The contrast between the two kinds of work certainly helped in the infantilizing of the patients. When Betty MacDonald asked her occupational-therapy instructor for permission to practice shorthand in lieu of crocheting, the response was hostile: "You're no better than the rest of us." And when, as an ambulent patient assigned to typing up and mimeographing the sanatorium magazine, MacDonald made the mistake of correcting the grammar and spelling of the contributions, she was rebuked.

For sanatorium writing was like sanatorium work; patients were encouraged to do it for their in-house organs but were strongly discouraged from aspiring to the tough professional prose Betty MacDonald produced in *The Plague and I*. Considering how widespread publicity about the sanatorium was and how many American families were directly affected by tuberculosis, it is curious to note how few patients wrote about the experience of sanatorium life for the general public. Write they did, and incessantly, but primarily for themselves, in a forum as isolated as their hospital lives and in a style that bore the same relation to literature as occupational therapy bore to manufacturing. They were sternly admonished not to get above themselves; in the decades of Eliot, Pound, and Laura Riding, sanatorium poetry (a genre much encouraged from patients, and apparently popular with them) remained rigidly sentimental, rooted firmly in children's verse:

> I love to lie on my sleeping porch
> And watch the clouds so high
> A shifting scene on an azure screen
> Make pictures in the sky.
>
> Six baby cloudlets go sailing by
> Then joining hands, I see
> Them gaily prance in a lilting dance
> Frolicking merrily.

The temptation to criticize such outpourings is strong, but misses something in that it overlooks the fact that most patients entered willingly into the hospital routine, after the initial ritual struggle; submitting themselves to authority, complaisantly returning to a kind of spiritual childhood, as if life might be relived from the beginning once again, and lost health thus restored. The sanatorium encouraged, perhaps demanded, the active participation of the patient, far more than most medical procedures do—the act alone of imagining yourself into the proper frame of mind seemed a real course of action, belying the apparent passivity etymologically latent in the very term "patient." Ironic detachment, perhaps preferable from a traditionally literary point of view, may not have been therapeutic: the patient was already debilitatingly detached from life by his illness, and further alienation on top of that might be dangerous. The doctors thought so, at least.

So did most patients. In 1955 the Firland Sanatorium, the hospital Betty MacDonald had entered some twenty years before, conducted a study of its patients' attitudes; overwhelmingly the respondents bought the hospital's image of them and itself: 89.5 percent thought Firland had helped them adjust to illness; 54.1 percent thought it a great help; 91.3 percent thought they would not get better care in another hospital;

92.3 percent reported that occupational therapy was an "important help" to them; only 24.4 percent reported themselves as often bored. So comforting and all-enveloping was the routine that discharged patients, even recalcitrant ones, often found readjustment to the world traumatic. Betty MacDonald recalled months during which she saw only ex-patients, gossiped compulsively about the Pines and its staff, and found the company of her family and nontubercular friends grating and alien. Saranac Lake and its environs still harbor a sizable population of ex-patients who, discharged, found themselves unable to tear themselves away from the community. The Trudeau Institute, successor of the Adirondack Cottage Sanatorium, still employs ex-patients and former staff, who remain attached to it out of affection for their days at the hospital. Isabel Smith, discharged, remained in Saranac until her death.

If on the one hand such behavior seems to constitute a flight from reality, and the typical sanatorium alumnus a social cripple, there was another side to it. The ex-patients had lived with the threat of hopelessness and death and had found a place that possibly conquered, and at least coped with, both. If life might look on the sanatorium as a colony of rootless exiles, the sanatorium could quietly look on life as a domain of false gods, ignoring the profound horrors with which the sanatorium had somehow learned to live. Saranac was a place that bore a burden the rest of the world rejected; it grew used to tourists speeding through with handkerchiefs clutched over their mouths. Its isolation may at times have made it seem naïve and childish, but it never lost sight of the childishness of a world that tried to ignore what the sanatorium faced. One recovered patient, the novelist Allan Seager, recalling his departure from Saranac, captures the double irony in a vignette on the railway platform that embodies the quizzical regard in which America and the sanatorium held each other.

> I felt there was a certain arrogance in my departure, in having plans beyond these mountains, in leaving at all because I left these friends behind. As we waited on the station platform for the train, feeling the involved ironies

of each other's good wishes, it was George who loosened us up. "Well, you won't be going alone," he said. I seemed to be. No other passengers were waiting. George pointed to two long pine boxes stacked one on top of the other at the end of the platform. It was funny then, desperate but funny, but only now do I see how courteous it was.

5

"The Burden of Human Misery, Not Its Own":
Saranac Lake

How little those who so often speak disparagingly of
Saranac Lake, because it harbors so many invalids, know
of the burden of human misery, not its own, which this
small and remote town has carried and ministered to as
best it could for so many years!
                    —EDWARD L. TRUDEAU, *An Autobiography*

In January of 1920, Saranac Lake was readying itself for Mid-
Winter Carnival. The ice company, guided by a local architect,
cut great blocks from the deep-frozen lake and dragged them
by horse-drawn sledge into the town center. There, volunteers
painstakingly assembled them—carelessness might precipitate
the whole fragile, fanciful pile into the street—and the Ice
Palace, at the time the only one in North America, rose above
the town, where, grandly illuminated, it would remain until
the spring thaw destroyed it.

At ten-thirty on the morning of January 27, the grand parade
began forming on Broadway, just south of the firehouse. To a
casual eye it might have looked like any small town's festive
gathering: the Marshall, Miss Kathryn Lavallee, led it, followed
by the newly crowned Carnival Queen and the Saranac Lake
Businessmen's Band. The Fire Department contributed a float
portraying Peace and Liberty, the W. C. Leonard Company
sponsored a Russian Sleigh, the Knights of Columbus marched
as Dixie Minstrels. There were a Horsemobile, a Chariot of
Jupiter, an Old Time Adirondack Hunting Camp; A. Fortune

and Company, the leading embalmer, displayed, perhaps inopportunely, "The Result of a Day's Hunt in the Adirondacks."

But a nearer glance at the parade would have discovered more exotic sights. "City of the Sick," one of Saranac's own newspapers had christened it, and its celebrations reflected its civic mission. The ill were not banished to the outlying sanatoriums; their presence was not ignored but rather publicized, even ceremonially emphasized. The Altavista Lodge, an expensive private sanatorium recently built within the city limits, sponsored a decorated float and manned it with ambulent patients. So did the Trudeau Sanatorium—its theme was "Gates A-Jar." The Associated Physicians of Saranac Lake appeared in a *tableau vivant* representing the Landing of the Pilgrims, while the Associated Pharmacies mounted a Living Carnival Poster, and the Red Cross paraded a giant Helping Hand. One year, on a sledge drawn by four white horses and festooned with an American flag and evergreen boughs stood a group of muffled, bundled, hatted and coated figures, new arrivals to the cure: "WE HAVE JUST COME FOR OUR HEALTH," their float announced.

The parade wound down Broadway to the shore of Lake Flower to the Riverside Inn, where most newly arriving patients stayed, and where they were met by the welcoming committee of the Anti-Tuberculosis Society. Then it turned up Church Street, passing the house where Edward Livingston Trudeau had died five years before (and where, half a century later, his grandson Frank was still practicing medicine), finally dispersing at Berkeley Square. In the festivities that followed, consumption branded no one; visitors and residents, doctors and patients, the healthy and the tubercular—all mixed indiscriminately. There was a fancy-dress skating carnival for adults that evening beneath the floodlit Ice Palace, and an indoor ball afterward. On Saturday there were sports competitions, more skating, another ball. Sunday the celebrations culminated with a grand finale, "The Storming and Defense of the Ice Palace," and a fireworks display. In between there were hayrides, trips on sleighs decorated with fresh flowers, costumes, flirtations, romances. Invalids, children, burghers, and visiting sports competitors trudged companionably through the hard-packed snow in the streets (plowing them had been given up as futile), their costumes sometimes fantastic but their footwear always sensible—three or four pairs of home-knit wool socks, shoes, and overshoes.

When one entered Saranac Lake for the first time, whether as a visitor or healthseeker, one might or might not notice the telltale signs of the way it earned its living. The larger sanatoriums, like the Trudeau, Ray Brook, Stony Wold, the National Variety Artists' Lodge (later the Will Rogers Memorial), and the Reception Hospital, were either outside town on their own substantial properties or hidden away on secondary thoroughfares. Main Street, Broadway, and Church Street resembled more or less exactly their counterparts in a hundred contemporary small American towns. But a closer look could, to the uninitiated, be unsettling. On any given day, a few somber wooden boxes might be seen waiting on the platform of the railway station, the newly dead on their way home along with the living. From two to four every afternoon, the streets fell eerily silent as patients and nonpatients alike observed rest hours; shops closed, deliveries ceased, children were shushed and herded indoors. Afterward, you might see the newly recovered tubercular and the nontubercular going about their business normally; but you might notice others, fledgling convalescents just off bed rest, gingerly taking their first half hour of exercise, timing themselves, as Lawrason Brown insisted, to the last second. When he had finished making rounds among his housebound tubercular patients, Dr. Francis B. Trudeau could, if he'd forgotten his gloves, be seen manipulating his steering wheel with his elbows, so as to avoid contamination. And then, since the cure was, after all, an outdoor life, one saw patients everywhere, lying motionless on innumerable porches in their cure chairs. That might seem reassuring, but it could also strike terror. "Oh God, Mikie, what's the use?" Helene McClintock asked her husband as, arriving to take the cure at the beginning of the Depression, the sight greeted her.

I know now, for the first time, that I'm sick. I'm like those people on the porches, sick. No matter how rotten I've felt, I have not known that until now. . . . But now I know it, know it clear through me, down into my feelings. I'm sick.

Saranac did its best to cushion its guests, its sick, and itself against the grim reality off which it lived, but the dark notes had a way of reasserting themselves. The Santanoni, the most expensive and luxurious private sanatorium, sent its dead downstairs in an elevator so discreetly small that the undertaker had to sit the corpses in his lap to get them out of the building. As far as possible, it reproduced the luxury of a first-class hotel, but a quiet uneasiness pervaded it nonetheless. Elizabeth Mooney, whose mother stayed there in the 1920s, sensed this on her first childhood visit to the sickroom:

It is a big room and she is wearing her marabou trimmed negligee and smiling at us. She has been sewing during the long hours of rest and holds up a little crepe-de-chine dress which has puff sleeves and smocking. I let loose of Father's hand and run to the bedside to take it while she holds it up to me, gauging the fit.

In the background I hear my father's voice. "Stand back," he says. "Don't get too close."

The temptation to gloom provoked in Saranac, as it had in the sanatorium movement, a countervailing determination to preserve good cheer at all costs. But here it became not merely a therapeutic fiction but a matter of civic pride, finding its way into the publicity issued by the Chamber of Commerce, and eventually becoming part of folk memories of the tuberculosis era. Nostalgia and affection are the dominant themes in the recollections of ex-patients and citizens who lived there before the Depression, and even afterward. It was lively, they insist, its optimism not merely brave pretense but the natural high spirits of a boom town. The sanatoriums were not merely hospitals or even sources of steady employment; they were thought of as cultural resources, and their frequent entertainments for patients and guests were regarded as public theatrical events, worthy of attention by local newspaper critics. One vaudeville evening at the Trudeau Sanatorium, "Microbial Merriment, Or, the Bassillies of 1925," was praised by the *Adirondack Enterprise,* Saranac's leading newspaper, as a "riot of fun."

A number of episodes made up the play, the first being "The Hallelujah San," supposedly a model sanatorium which really succeeded in being everything a sanatorium should not be. "Dark Doings on the Cousinola" depicted the adventures of a Trudeau couple caught out after hours. "Dr. Green's Question Box," a travesty on the Wednesday noon question box instituted by Dr. Lawrason Brown, was packed with apt quips and proved an instant hit.

Veterans remember the life not as grotesque but as "wonderful, . . . beautiful." Bill McLaughlin, later to become a fixture in Saranac political life, entered the Trudeau in 1939, and though he remained for his entire stay in Ludington, the sometimes-dreaded infirmary, he afterward remembered having "as much fun there" as other patients did in the freer atmosphere of the residential cottages. There were flirtations and romances with the new crop of student nurses who arrived each six or eight weeks, and a patient population mainly young and often well educated—"no duds . . . like a hotel, really. . . . We all looked better than anybody coming to visit us."

Saranac in the 1920s also supported a roaring trade in contraband Canadian liquor smuggled southward through the Adirondacks, and the fruits of that commerce buoyed up the spirits of the sick and boosted the local economy. Illness brought the rich and famous, who built lavish single-family cure residences on the select streets; the Trudeau, as the nation's leading sanatorium, was a magnet for young doctors either stricken with the disease or interested in treating it.

131

William Morris, who kept a summer camp nearby, helped found the National Variety Artists' Lodge, a sanatorium for performers, which brought an influx of musicians, actors, and writers. Stores throve, new businesses opened, the population grew, and by the late 1920s the town fathers were envisioning a brilliant future for themselves—at one point there was even a streetcar system on the drawing board. If prosperity built itself on the sufferings of the ill, at least its benefits helped raise their spirits. They knew, and the town freely admitted, that they were the cause and the guarantors of it. Esther Mirick remembered Saranac in the twenties as "completely run for the sick people"; the school system, for which she worked, accommodated three hundred to four hundred children from invalid families. Volunteers met the sick as they alit at the station and directed them to the sanatoriums or the 1,300-odd beds available in privately run cure cottages. Saranac Lake was a town shaped by tuberculosis as Chicago was shaped by railroads—its history, its appearance, and its customs defined by its mission.

Its story was, even by American standards, a short one. The bustling Saranac Lake of the twenties was the work of a single generation, though its history as a forlorn outpost went back much farther. The first white settler, Jacob Moody, arrived in 1819, followed by one Captain Pliny Miller, who built a dam and sawmill on the site of what later became the Riverside Inn. A few small hunting lodges appeared; nearby Paul Smith began to attract his gilded patrons. They so took to the life that they began buying up huge tracts of wilderness and building immense pseudorustic retreats for summer residence. "When [Smith] came into the Adirondacks to found his little hostelry," as Francis Trudeau puts it, "the woods were full of Indians. When he left they were full of millionaires."

Still, growth came slowly. By 1880 about three hundred souls were living there but in primitive isolation, for the outside world remained remote and travel arduous. The departing visitor or native bound for civilization boarded a stage, which lurched along rudimentary roads for thirty-two miles, through Bloomingdale and Franklin Falls, to Ausable. There he transferred to the narrow-gauge Chateaugay Railway, which disgorged him at Plattsburgh and enabled him to switch to the main-line railroads, north to Canada or south to Albany and New York. "The Adirondack Mountains, as Dr. Trudeau found them," the *Enterprise* wrote in its 1915 memorial issue, "might have been termed the Great Inaccessible, or the Other Side of Beyond." Nonetheless, spurred by rumor, medical opinion, or Alfred Loomis's 1879 article in the *Medical Record,* "The Adirondack Region as a Therapeutical Agent in the Treatment of Pulmonary Tuberculosis," invalids began to trickle into the region and to attach themselves to Trudeau. Considering how steeped in local myth these early healthseek-ers are, we know little about them. Trudeau never made it quite clear in *An Autobiography* just how or when he began to formulate the cure; in the early years he and Loomis both frankly admitted ignorance as to why the Adirondacks worked their health-giving effect: "Here . . . there is every inducement for one to lead an out-of-door life; the very surroundings infuse new life into the feeble body, and one daily grows stronger and stronger and feels better, scarcely able to tell how or why."

By 1885 the trickle of invalids had become a steady flow, whom the natives appear to have welcomed unthinkingly, as no more exotic than the merchant princes who descended on Paul Smith each summer in search of unsuspecting deer and bear. When the Little Red opened that year, the two working women who came to recuperate in it can scarcely have seemed like the vanguard of an invasion; local farmers and their wives readily took on necessary tasks like cooking, housekeeping, and nursing. The patients simply soaked up the rigors and pleasures of the wilderness, for, despite the example of Breh-mer and Dettweiler, Trudeau trusted to serendipity and the mountains, counting on a therapeutic effect. In contrast with the finical timetables later prescribed by Lawrason Brown, Trudeau's early patients simply lived in the wilderness, rest-ing. Carolyn Pentland Lindsay came in 1887.

My sister and I were assigned to the "Little Red" Cottage, the first one, built in 1884. . . . Things were not altogether ideal then. . . . The water system was not adequate; sputum cups in the present form were not used. Time hung heavily, as the village of Saranac Lake had only a few houses, a saw mill, a post office and store, so there was no entertainment of any kind. The daily ride in winter wrapped in fur coats and with hot bricks at the feet, was almost a dissipation; and the arrival of the stage with the mail and a possible express package was excitement enough to cause a run of fever. The childish amusements we indulged in would make a 1924 patient smile: splitting birch bark, stripping balsam, sliding and coasting, gathering spruce gum, and in the spring gathering the most beautiful mountain violets, picking wild strawberries and later marvelous blueberries.

Photographs of these earliest patients, engaged in relatively normal activities, contrast markedly with the later portraits, in which rows of supine figures stretch into the distance, lying on porches in identical cure chairs and lap robes, staring off at the mountains. But Mrs. Lindsay's improvised regimen seems to have worked for her: in 1925 she was still not only alive but flourishing, working in Albany as superintendent of the Woman's Christian Temperance Union's department of exhibits and fairs.

By 1890 there were about twenty-five patients at the Adirondack Cottage Sanatorium. The Little Red had been joined by new cottages, the Little Blue and the Little Green. Board was five dollars a week, and though conditions were still rough-and-ready, Trudeau was a conscientious doctor, not content to rest on successes that might, after all, have been luck. He taught himself bacteriology and, following Robert Koch, began a course of experiments with the tubercle bacillus in his own laboratory; he tested new, and sometimes exotic, therapies as they were touted in medical journals. Mrs. Lindsay remembered being ordered at one point to sing and whistle; at another, to inhale hydrogen sulfide gas; at still another, to breathe a medicated oxygen as she "sat shut up in a glass cabinet for a stated period weekly." Shortly after the advent of Koch's lymph (the celebrated "cure" announced in 1890 by the discoverer of the tubercle bacillus), a sample arrived at Saranac, and though Trudeau was skeptical about it from the outset, he continued experimenting with it for the rest of his life. Miss Emeline Cooper, a patient at the sanatorium in 1893, took the treatment: "For nine months I had daily injections and I was looked upon as a very fine and satisfactory result."

Toward the turn of the twentieth century the number of patients had grown again, and the cure turned from an informal and accidental routine into the bedrock of Saranac's village life. Publicity, initially confined to the medical press and conveyed to invalids through their physicians, began to make its way into mass-circulation journals, and in 1898 Saranac merited an article in the *New York Evening Post*. The sanatorium had grown, becoming a magnet for philanthropy, and the village was beginning to view the onslaught of patients both as a challenge and a source of potential growth and prosperity. The cure was beginning to take the shape it kept throughout the rest of its history:

> There are about 100 invalids cared for at the sanitarium and many poor applicants have to be turned away; but many other hundreds are scattered about throughout an area of a thousand or two square miles. All along the highways of the region can be seen figures bundled and wrapped, sitting on piazzas, "taking the cure," or "chewing air," as it is termed by the invalids. The old theory that a great deal of exercise is beneficial to those suffering from tuberculosis has been modified; in fact it has been abandoned in cases where there is any evidence of active trouble from the disease. . . .

Communication with the outside world became easier when, in 1888, the Chateaugay Railway finally came to Saranac. The village was incorporated in 1892, with Trudeau as its first president. Its first town budget was a modest $500, but the population had tripled from the pretubercular era to about 1,200, and by 1893 sewer and water systems were under construction. Streets were paved, and soon thereafter builders and businessmen endowed their mountain hamlet with urban ambitions. The scale was miniature, but the feeling unmistakably citified: "City of the Sick," the publicity phrase coined by a local paper, was to prove truer than its originator hoped. For as it grew, Saranac's mission as a health center imposed on it an order and coherence foreign to its straggling rival towns. The ill, after all, couldn't walk far; they needed a wide variety of services that had to be delivered to them as efficiently as possible. As a result the town adopted the passion for planning that originated with Brehmer and that became a fixture of the sanatorium movement, with its fondness for a harmonious mix of the functional and the pleasing, the efficient and the relaxed.

Even today, in its depressed state and despite empty storefronts and the conversion of the sanatoriums into jails, offices, and conference centers, Saranac retains an energetic and thoroughly urban air. Because they required so much land, the major sanatoriums were built away from the town center, and yet were not quite hidden, so that, as you drive in, they serve as a transition from the outlying wilderness to the activity of the village. Ray Brook Sanatorium, now a prison, lies to the east on the road from Lake Placid; the Trudeau Sanatorium, just outside to the north. (It now serves as headquarters for the American Management Institute.) You then pass through the residential streets, spacious and lined with former private sanatoriums, and reach a compact downtown, a felicitous miniature potpourri of city themes. Main Street is straight and level; Broadway, curved and hilly, crossing the Saranac River, which runs through the center of town, closely bordered by buildings with overhanging porches. Broadway and Main converge at an unmistakable center, Berkeley Square, from which you can look down to the river, across to the leading hotel and Edward Livingston Trudeau's old home, or southward to a park on the shore of Lake Flower. Broadway and Main Street are built up, lined with early-twentieth-century two- and three-story brick buildings, engaging examples of bygone small-town grandiosity. But the surrounding thoroughfares are full of green space, lined by modest buildings that, visible from Berkeley Square, soften the impression conveyed by the business district and modulate it smoothly into the residential streets. The shops reveal a place lived in, not merely visited or limited to supplying the needs of outlying farms: clothing, furniture, five-and-ten, books, hardware, pharmacy, coffee shop, bakery, bar, rooming house, news dealer, hotel.

Compare Lake Placid, Saranac's near neighbor and arch rival. (An old story traces this to an immemorial intervillage football game that Saranac won by a score of 102–0.) Placid, despite the Olympics and a comparatively healthy tourist economy, sprawls haphazardly along Mirror Lake and below. There is little sense of center, none of urban energy, and most of the businesses are blatantly ephemeral tourist traps—McDonald's, Custard Mustard 'n' Brew, Steak 'n' Burger, the Alpine Mall, and the Handlebar (dispensing Discount Liquor, Camping Information, Cold Six-Packs, Ice, Kegs, Sandwiches, and Homemade Chili, as well as housing a Historical Museum). Whatever the sadness of its current depressed state, Saranac lacks such bumptious frivolity; it retains the completeness, the balance, and even some of the vitality its mission invested it with.

Nor is it simply in its town plan that Saranac inherited from tuberculosis a unique appearance; over the decades of its growth, it engendered a new style of domestic architecture, adapted to the requirements of the cure, and in time this transformed the appearance of the residential streets. When growth commenced in the 1880s the town began to build houses much like those in any contemporary village of comparable size: Queen Anne cottages of balloon construction, informal and pleasingly irregular in floor plan, often capped by jutting asymmetrical gables and festooned with verandas. But when the ill began to arrive in force, and as the cure, under Lawrason Brown's influence, came to demand long hours outdoors under protection from inclement weather, these cottages began to evolve. The Trudeau Sanatorium and its sister institutions couldn't accommodate all the applicants who descended on Saranac Lake hoping for admission; some were too ill, others not ill enough, still others for one reason or another not suited to institutional life. In response, and sensing an economic opportunity, the townspeople began to take in boarders, supplying nursing care and tray service for the bed-ridden; by 1930 the "cure cottage" had become a mainstay of the local economy and a principle of architecture. For Saranac houses began to acquire a distinctive shape. Formerly well supplied with outdoor porches, they now bristled with them.

Often these were tacked on wherever they fit, when a for-mer private residence became a private sanatorium. If the owners attracted the tubercular and made a success of their enterprise, new porches would sprout above or beside old ones; houses sprawled outward, acquiring facades of glass. Eventually local architects began designing buildings explic-itly to the requirements of the cure, and the results gave Sara-nac a unique urban profile. Ubiquitous porches blurred or even hid the building lines, and houses became in conse-quence rather shapeless but buxom, even maternal, and pleas-antly informal. As they expanded, they also grew toward each other and toward the street, overcoming the isolation and in-wardness implicit in the wide lawns and dense shrubbery com-mon in American towns. The invalid was confined to his porch; it was his main contact with the world as well as the instrument of his therapy. And in Saranac these porches, visible every-where and pushed by growth into companionable contact with each other, became an amenity of village life. From them you might stare off at Mount Pisgah or Lake Flower, but you might also chat with a fellow consumptive or a schoolchild passing on the street. Adelaide Crapsey's cure cottage fronted on a ceme-tery, but that depressing vista was unusual for Saranac, though useful for Crapsey since she was a poet and the sight inspired perhaps her best poem, "To the Dead in the Grave-Yard under My Window." Normally the Saranac porch was not a lonely aerie but a social force, allowing privacy but encouraging com-munication, and it became an obligatory feature of every building in the town, commercial as well as domestic.

Perhaps the quintessential Saranac cure home was the Blauvelt Cottage at 16 Helen Street (or Hemorrhage Hill, as patients dubbed it; it rises steeply from Church Street near the
Trudeau house, and climbing it was a challenge for the shaky
invalid commencing exercise). Its owner, Mrs. B. H. Adams,
advertised its virtues in 1907.

> Situated on the summit of Helen Street Hill is the Blauvelt
> Cottage, affording a view of the village that is at once
> picturesque and superb. Large, newly and pleasantly fur-
> nished rooms with all modern improvements, hot water
> heat and electric light. Beds of best quality. The table and
> service is unexcelled. Rates $15 per week and upwards.
> For further particulars address Mrs. B. H. Adams. . . .

Phil Gallos, in his excellent history, *Cure Cottages of Saranac
Lake,* recorded the story of this cottage since it was built in
approximately 1898. In the earliest surviving pictures, the
Blauvelt Cottage is a conventional Queen Anne house, with
the typical irregular floor plan, jutting wings, large windows,
dormers, and a sweeping veranda, partly glassed in and appropriate for sitting out. In later photographs, the house balloons
outward, acquiring more dormers and new porches (eventually six of the latter), and the house, though it has lost most of
its Queen Anne character, has gained a homely and genial
comfort. It's massive, yet because of its glass, also light; imposing, but thanks to the apparent improvisation, also informal;
less bungalowlike and so indefinably more urban, though not
in any conventional urban mode. In growing upward and outward, the house and its neighbors have engaged themselves
more intimately with each other and with the street; houses
that otherwise would have turned inward on themselves, con-
cealed by trees and spacious lots, form a continuous street-
scape, communicating with each other and the thoroughfare
through their porches.

Saranac's urban profile was very much its own, and very
much an expression of the cure. For the cure was communal,
and in that sense urban, but, developed and sophisticated an

arrangement though the sanatorium was, it also preserved the illusion of being rural. Saranac's town houses were country houses grown up and grown together. And their style was not without influence. By the 1920s the sleeping porch, under the influence of the national antituberculosis crusade, had become a fixture of American middle-class house design. The movement had asserted that sleeping out was not only an essential part of the cure but a health-giving and pleasant practice for the tubercular and nontubercular alike. George F. Babbitt's Dutch Colonial house in Zenith has a sleeping porch—what more conclusive sign that it had leapt from the tubercular fringe into the mid-American mainstream?

The townspeople soon realized their streets and buildings were a composition as well as a chance gathering, and became careful about preserving the town's appearance. What may have begun out of a natural care for public health quickly translated itself into a preoccupation with aesthetics; in the great days, after all, it became accustomed to celebrities. Robert Louis Stevenson, coming in 1887 to take the cure (in fact he appears to have suffered not from consumption but from chronic bronchitis), was the first but by no means the last: Ralph Waldo Emerson, Ernest Hemingway, John Dos Passos, Edna Ferber, Marjorie Merriweather Post—all lived nearby, summered nearby, or took the cure in one or more of its available forms. Calvin Coolidge vacationed on nearby Lake Osgood; and Al Smith visited him there in July 1926. "Slightly delayed on their scheduled automobile trip to Paul Smith's," the *Enterprise* drily noted, "the Governor's party passed through Saranac Lake at 10:45 today at high speed. The entourage swept into Main Street from River Street at a fast clip, with two brown uniformed motor vehicle inspectors on a motorcycle clearing traffic."

Perhaps the celebrities passed through quickly and unheedingly, but they came nonetheless. Consumption had made the town grow, had made it prosperous, had made it famous, and that in a region noted for its poverty and backwardness as much as for its natural beauty. In prospect the history of a town so constituted would seem parasitic, even ghoulish, as if battening on misfortune to profit from it. But in fact, and allowing for the distortions of nostalgia and for a town's natural desire to present itself to the world in the best possible light, the very reverse seems to have been the case. Saranac in its heyday was an object lesson in how to live with a fatal disease, not denying it, yet not succumbing to it. The consumptive weren't oppressed or discriminated against, but neither were they coddled; Saranac adapted its normal life to them, and they adapted, more gradually and hesitantly, to it. The sick and the well lived in a miniature world acceptable to both. The streets emptied from two to four in the afternoon for rest period; but in the evening the Pontiac Theatre filled with the tubercular and the nontubercular alike. Healthy and ill, the citizens may well have been haunted by the solemn bourdon that sounded persistently underneath daily life, but they collaborated in building a city on a singular and admirable principle, the normalization of mortal illness without the trivialization of it.

In the 1906 Adirondack directory there was already evidence of a subtle and tacit concordat between the well and the ill. Invalids were listed exactly as were the permanent residents, except for a discreet notation that they were "boarding" at their designated addresses; thus they were marked, yet not ostracized. For its modest population of 4,000 (triple the incorporation year of 1892), Saranac boasted a disproportionately large number of service businesses: the ill needed things that otherwise might surface only in the luxury-hungry economy of a large city. Ernest Grice, "The Hustling Newspaper Boy," promised to deliver out-of-town newspapers by hand within twenty minutes of their arrival at the station. In 1910 Charles F. Pasho, the leading barber, gave up his shop to make "cottage calls exclusively. . . . All implements," Pasho warranted, "are sterilized and kept in a perfectly sanitary condition." Foy's Theatre, at 45 Broadway, besides promising its patrons first-rate entertainment, also offered reassurance. "Sanitary— Clean—Healthful . . . the only amusement house in town that is regularly disinfected by the Board of Health." One local

141

irony, and a source of grim amusement to the invalids (or healthseekers, as Saranac called them), was A. Fortune and Co., a many-tentacled family business (still in existence) that, in addition to manufacturing the most popular brand of Adirondack cure chair and selling "bedding, carpets, tapestries, window shades, etc.," as well as children's sleds, served in 1906 as Saranac's only embalmer. But the latter business was handled delicately. Look up "embalmer" in the directory and you were referred to Fortune's advertisement, which, however, mentioned only its more cheerful services.

The array of businesses that arose as the town grew throughout the early years of the century is also telling. In 1906 there were, apart from the Adirondack Cottage Sanatorium and outlying hospitals (the Sanatorium Gabriels, for example, was opened by the Sisters of Mercy in 1897 and was the first to admit black patients), seventeen cure cottages listed in the directory. There were also four druggists, who became all-purpose service agents, delivering everything from postage stamps to bootleg liquor (in baby bottles). There were eight liveries in town, three dairies (this was the period during which invalids were encouraged to drink large quantities of milk), and eleven physicians in private practice. (Others, of course, were exclusively engaged to treat patients at the large sanatoriums.)

Perhaps the zenith year for Saranac Lake was 1930. The population had peaked at 8,020; and the board of trustees estimated that one hundred thousand visitors passed through town yearly. The community now could boast thirteen druggists, five undertakers, fifty-three private physicians, thirteen private-duty nurses, seven churches, two banks, a savings and loan association, four hotels, two apartment hotels, and nineteen taxi services. The town assessed the value of its buildings—which featured a new town hall and a first-class theater—at a total of $8 million. There were six major sanatoriums, 150 private cure cottages, and the well-equipped Saranac Lake General Hospital. Not long after, a civic airport opened at nearby Lake Clear, and boosters were promoting the construction of another state hospital to supplement the facility at Ray Brook. "Health-seekers feel that they definitely 'belong' here, that they are members of a community which understands them and takes them unto itself," one flyer assured the prospective newcomer; others reassured vacationers. "There should be no confusion," a 1932 Chamber of Commerce brochure insisted, "as to the advisability of having both the Health Seeker and Recreationist on one basis. Are they not the same issue—one trying to regain what he has lost, the other trying to preserve that which he has?"

Tact and discretion intertwined with puffery, and commercial life adjusted itself accordingly. Receptive businesses subtly assured consumptives that their special needs would be accommodated, but without treading on their sensibilities. "MARCELLING *as it should be done,*" the Sullivan Beauty Shoppe promised in large type, then adding, for the benefit of those still on restricted exercise, "The Only Beauty Parlor in Town on the Ground Floor." And although the Hotel Saranac, built in 1926, may have meant to discourage the tubercular by putting its lobby on the second floor, as a rule Saranac Lake, in the face of widespread phthisophobia, demonstrated a strong sense of public conscience.

Its disproportionately large medical fraternity soon became an active presence in public life. Not only had Edward Livingston Trudeau been the first president of the incorporated village; Edward R. Baldwin, the superintendent at Trudeau during the twenties and thirties, took as keen an interest in the politics of the town as he did in the medical affairs of the sanatorium, working with the Chamber of Commerce, collecting pamphlets on the town's history, and serving on its relief committee during the Depression. In 1907 the local physicians, led by the indefatigable Lawrason Brown, formed a local antituberculosis society, which became both a monitor of health conditions and a referral service for healthseekers. The effort was purely voluntary, but, as its 1931 annual report suggests, it became a significant force in the community.

The Saranac Lake Society for the Control of Tuberculosis was organized . . . to meet problems of vital importance to the Adirondack region and to safeguard and benefit the community of Saranac Lake:

1. By educating the people in regard to the proper sanitary measures in relation to tuberculosis by lectures, the distribution of literature, and other appropriate means.

2. By aiding the Board of Health in bringing home to the people the necessity of enforcing these measures, especially such as deal with expectoration and disinfection.

3. By encouraging and assisting all hotels and boarding houses to enforce these measures.

4. By discouraging the sending to the Adirondacks of hopelessly ill persons who are without means of support.

5. By maintaining a Free Bureau of Information for health-seekers, with [some of] the following objects: (a) to furnish reliable and impartial information concerning the conditions and cost of living in Saranac Lake and vicinity; (b) to explain the conditions under which admission to various semicharitable and private institutions is to be gained; (c) to investigate needy cases and provide temporary aid or nursing when necessary; [and] to cooperate with the Chamber of Commerce and business interests in distributing suitable literature.

New patients were taken from the station to the Riverside Inn, and given a physical examination to assess their condition. Those not immediately bound for a sanatorium were given a list of boarding cottages in appropriate price ranges and supplied with an itinerary so they could visit their prospective quarters in the least tiring order.

"My own idea about advertising the village," Dr. Baldwin wrote to a colleague in 1935, "is that it should be constantly kept before the public as a health [and] pleasure resort having unusual facilities and sanitary control." Sickness and death were thus firmly woven into the tissue of the town's daily life; how well this worked is illustrated no better than by the shock and incredulity with which it greeted the occasional tragedies to which, given its stock in trade, one would have thought it inured and resigned.

The Burden of Human Misery, Not Its Own

On January 16, 1907, Miss Helen Higbey, a Utica nurse curing at Saranac, died of a self-administered overdose of acetanilid. The *Northern New Yorker* reported the death under a prominent headline, but the purpose of the story was reassurance rather than sensationalism. The death, the paper implausibly but soothingly announced, was "clearly one of an accidental nature," so "there was no necessity for an inquest": apparently a town inured to the White Plague panicked at the hint of suicide. And in a famous 1930 incident still remembered by the village's older residents, a woman lay down on the railroad tracks and waited patiently for an incoming train to run over her. The incident caused a furor, for intrusions of melodrama, of histrionic despair, were unwelcome. "Being told we have tuberculosis," the town board of trustees wrote in 1935 to prospective patients, "is always a shock, because it crept up on us like a thief in the dark, and when we were well." But Saranac Lake prided itself on not letting the violence of the shock disarrange life more than was necessary. "You will feel at home. Your selection of a place to live will not be restricted to one section, which makes Saranac Lake unique as a health resort."

With so much economically invested in sustaining such a public image, Saranac was understandably sensitive about the way the nation saw it, alert to any criticism. A 1926 feature in the Philadelphia *Public Ledger* that (among other things) called the town's tubercular residents "poor suffering mortals carrying the smile of hope" and the typical patients "people of small means who board in the town or are patients of the Adirondack Cottage Sanatorium" outraged Saranackers and provoked a hot retort in the *Enterprise*. Yet the *Ledger* had said nothing the town hadn't already said about itself. In the closing pages of *An Autobiography*, Edward Livingston Trudeau wrote virtually the same thing:

> How little those who so often speak disparagingly of Saranac Lake, because it harbors so many invalids, know of the burden of human misery, not its own, which this small and remote town has carried and ministered to as best it could for so many years! The selfishness, cruelty or stupidity of

145

terror-stricken relatives and friends which urges a poor
and hopelessly ill consumptive, without money, to come
to die in so remote a region, among strangers, only adds
loneliness and many discomforts to his unfortunate lot,
and an additional burden to the ever over-taxed charity
of the town.

But an outsider making the same observation was impermissi-
ble. Saranac wanted to be known as a health resort, but at the
same time wanted no part of the ambiguity inevitable in a
more analytical and detached evaluation.

As Saranac was approaching the zenith of its years of prosperity, the local and the New York boards of health commis-
sioned a study to determine whether the concentration of
invalids had increased the incidence of tuberculosis among the
native population. But Forrest B. Ames, who conducted the
survey from May to September of 1917, had broader curiosi-
ties—he wanted to know how Saranac's special mission had
affected the social fabric of the village, and his conclusions,
published the following year in the *American Review of Tuberculosis,* form a picture of a town like no other.

At the time, Ames estimated, approximately 20 percent of
the 6,000 people living there had either active tuberculosis or
a past history of the disease. Among these, he counted 860
"transients," people curing in Saranac but not thinking of
themselves as residents, and 441 "permanents," people who
had first come for reasons of health but who had decided to
settle there for good. The numbers tell us something about
Saranac's channels of connection with the outside world—a
steady influx of immigrants, roughly half of whom stayed,
while the other half either died or went back home. Taken
together, the tubercular were a decided minority, yet also a
critical mass, a group large enough to be a force in the social
and political life of the town.

Curiously, though, the native population, the original stock,
turned out to show a far lower than expected incidence of
tuberculosis. Among them there were, in 1917, only four cases,

less than a third of a percent of the total in the town. Both morbidity and mortality among the natives was well below what would normally be seen in a population of its size. In part, this statistic may simply have been a result of tuberculosis consciousness: everyone knew how it was transmitted, and civic ordinances controlling dangerous behavior—spitting, for instance—were carefully enforced. And thanks to the Society for the Control of Tuberculosis, the sanatoriums, and the omnipresence of informed medical supervision, those afflicted with the disease were well educated against behavior that might spread contagion.

But it went beyond that. The very prosperity that came from consumption protected the town against it, an irony that Ames records even if he was unaware of it:

Saranac Lake is a closely built village. . . . Because of the short growing season agriculture is not generally followed. To favor good living conditions may be cited the fact that in the village are few instances of extreme poverty, the majority of families belonging to the moderately well-to-do class. Industrial occupations involving indoor work are few. The general intelligence of the people on subjects relating to tuberculosis is very high. Open air sports are common, for instance, boating, hunting, fishing, skating, etc.

Of course, the relative health of the natives (they also suffered from a lower-than-normal incidence of other epidemic diseases) served further to separate them from the sick—paradoxically, in a town devoted to the sick, and notably devoid of prejudice toward them, they were more definitively isolated from the healthy than they might have been elsewhere.

At approximately the same time that Saranac was being surveyed, the national association was inaugurating an experimental tuberculosis-control program in Framingham, Massachusetts. Part of the program included examinations of schoolchildren: 119 were inspected and, more or less simultaneously, 137 children underwent examinations in Saranac Lake. The results were significant. Eighty-two of the 119 Framingham children had enlarged tonsils and lymph nodes; only 17 of the 137 Saranac children did. Fourteen Framingham children had acute colds; 8 Saranac children did. Eleven Framingham children exhibited breathing abnormalities, against only 1 Saranac child. Framingham was by no means a particularly poor or unhealthy place—it had been chosen for a demonstration project because it was average. By contrast Saranac enjoyed, thanks both to its health awareness and the prosperity tuberculosis brought it, better-than-average living conditions, for the tubercular and the nontubercular alike. Among the invalids Ames interviewed, 38 were living in hotels, 174 in boardinghouses, 237 in private accommodations. Of these, Ames judged that a large majority were living in good or fair conditions.

However marked they may have been by illness, the tubercular were not discriminated against, at least not ostentatiously. Of the people Ames talked to who had ceased actively curing but who had chosen to remain in Saranac, 63 percent were working full-time; less than a quarter were completely idle. Of those able to work, a majority of those willing to divulge their incomes admitted to earning less than they had before they became ill; yet a significant percentage reported that they were earning as much as or more than they had made before moving to Saranac Lake.

Of course, occupations changed to suit the healthseeker's new habits and the mores of his new home. Twenty of the 285 ex-tubercular became boardinghouse proprietors, though none had earned a living this way before arriving in Saranac, and twenty-five were nurses, though only seventeen had followed that career before. Work for the others as well gradually shaped itself around the cure, as had their cultural and social lives. As early pioneers of the sanatorium movement had predicted, convalescent patients were drawn magnetically to the life of the cure and preferred to remain in touch with it when they were well. To the sympathetic observer, this integration of the healthy, the ill, and the once-ill in a happy and self-

sufficient community could seem a golden world, even a pre-
scriptive social model and a vision for the future.

But then the Depression struck. For Saranac Lake economic
stagnation was doubly devastating, since it coincided with eb-
bing morbidity and mortality from tuberculosis. The supply of
healthseekers dwindled; empty beds began appearing in the
sanatoriums and the Reception Hospital, and owners of cure
cottages began scrounging for patrons. Prohibition ended and
the bootlegging trade, now subsiding, deprived Saranac of
both color and cash. At first gradually, but then precipitously,
with the advent of antibiotic therapy in the late 1940s, Saranac
slid into a decline. "Everything was humming right along," Bill
McLaughlin remembers, but then "the bottom dropped out."
The well went home and the sick ceased to arrive.

Perhaps nothing brackets the rise and fall of Saranac so well
as the Reception Hospital, a charitable institution presided
over from its founding in 1902 to its closing in 1949 by a single
imposing figure, Miss Mary Prescott. Miss Prescott had come
to cure in Saranac Lake from her home in Massachusetts toward the end of the nineteenth century; by 1902 she was
sufficiently improved to begin to take an active interest in the
cure as a philanthropist. Already Saranac was burdened by the
arrival of destitute invalids ineligible for admission to the Adirondack Cottage Sanatorium and unable to find accommoda-
tion elsewhere. Miss Prescott, contributing her own funds and
soliciting more from friends and acquaintances, purchased a
house at 5 Franklin Avenue, "instituted for," she wrote in her
first annual report, "the benefit of those people who, coming
to Saranac Lake in search of health, find themselves alone and
discouraged, too ill to take care of themselves, and unable to
afford the expense of a private nurse and her board."

In 1902, the first year of its operation, the house, dubbed the
"Reception Hospital," took in thirty-seven patients. They
stayed an average of two months before departing for longer-
term accommodations; the total operating cost of the house
was $5,603.46.

By 1905 the hospital had expanded considerably, occupying
a new building on Helen Hill, built at a cost of $27,000; fifty-

seven patients were admitted during the course of the year, and sixty-nine were discharged. (There was also a waiting list for admission.) The peak year, however, was 1925, when the hospital admitted ninety-seven patients and discharged ninety-eight, keeping them at an average cost of $22.62 per patient per week and charging them (where they could pay so much) $14 a week for board. Helene McClintock stayed there after her initial period of floating from boardinghouse to boardinghouse, at the same time her husband Marshall gained admission at the Trudeau. Both found the conditions similarly pleasant—to move from a boarding cottage to any of the town institutions was, at least for patients of small means, a notable graduation. The care was more consistent and more professional, less subject to the vagaries of a boardinghouse keeper's moods, and there was more company.

Year after year Miss Prescott continued to keep the hospital; but beginning in the 1930s, like Saranac itself, it began to decline. Costs went down during the Depression, but so did admissions. The waiting list shrank; by the end of the 1930s it had disappeared, and vacancies were occurring. Patients, no more under pressure to leave to make room for newer patients, began to stay longer. Numbers dwindled, plunging from fifty-six in 1933 to twenty-six in 1941. By 1945, still well before the advent of antibiotics, Miss Prescott was in doubt about the future: "For yet another year Prescott House has been kept open, though sometimes it has seemed impossible." In 1949 it finally closed, having spanned virtually the whole history of the cure.

In October of that year the building went to the Study and Craft Guild, organized in the 1930s to give bedridden and convalescing patients instructions in various useful and/or time-killing occupations, a mobile version of the occupational therapy conducted in the institutional sanatoriums. But the craft guild itself was already turning into a general studies school for the whole community, fated to change as tuberculosis ebbed. Today the Reception Hospital still stands, but as an apartment house.

Much else has changed as well. Today there are but four druggists (they call themselves "pharmacies") and two undertakers (they call themselves "funeral directors," but A. Fortune is among them, having given up furniture, draperies, cure chairs, and sleds). There is only one taxi service, and twenty-four physicians. The town makes its living from prisons (into which, over the years, a number of the surrounding sanatoriums were transformed), from the Adirondack offices of the state department of environmental conservation; from two junior colleges; and from the Trudeau Institute, an immunological research laboratory and the sanatorium's successor. Saranac is hardly destitute, but its great days are over and the town knows it. There are empty storefronts; the Hotel Saranac is run as a training facility for students majoring in hotel management at a local college.

Those who remember the sanatorium era are fewer and fewer, mostly in their sixties, seventies, and eighties. Francis Trudeau, Edward Livingston Trudeau's grandson, practiced general medicine in Saranac, beginning his professional career just as the last patients were leaving. He became specially interested in sports medicine, and retired last year, evidently the last in an unbroken tradition of medical Trudeaus: his son, Garry, draws "Doonesbury." Saranac has not forgotten its past; far from it—signs on the outskirts of the town still welcome you to America's "Pioneer Health Resort," and the library assiduously collects memorabilia from the sanatorium era and oral-history records from survivors of it.

Bypassed by history though it was, it retains, compared to the garish opportunism of Lake Placid, an unassailable dignity. Even a cursory visit reveals it as a *place,* perhaps with little confidence in its present or future, but molded fatefully and uniquely by its past, dignified if disconsolate.

6

"Fewer and Better Doctors":
Tuberculosis and the Medical Profession

The improvement of medical education cannot . . . be
resisted on the ground that it will destroy schools and
restrict output: that is precisely what is needed. . . . The
country needs fewer and better doctors.
—ABRAHAM FLEXNER, *Medical
Education in the United States
and Canada* (1910)

Toward the end of the 1800s the medical profession was growing—so fast and so uncontrollably, in fact, that doctors who
paid attention to the situation were becoming frightened for
the future of their calling. In 1850 the United States had fifty-
two medical schools; by 1900 there were 160. Between 1870
and 1910 the general population grew by 138 percent, while
the number of physicians grew by 153 percent. They offered
a bewildering variety of medical regimens, from homeopathy
to Thomsonianism (a long-lived medical sect whose practitioners relied heavily on violent emetics), and the training they
underwent ranged from the rudimentary to the lunatic. As late
as the 1860s most medical schools, many of them money-mak-
ing enterprises, accepted anyone who wandered in off the
street, and even those destined for greatness were at this point
in their history very humble affairs. When Trudeau enrolled in
the College of Physicians and Surgeons in New York, it shared
a modest three-story brick building on the corner of Twenty-
third Street and Fourth Avenue with a drugstore and an ice
cream parlor. And the curriculum was correspondingly simple.

There was no entrance examination. All the student had to do was to matriculate at the college and pay a fee of five dollars, attend two or more courses of lectures at the college, and pass the very brief oral examinations which each professor gave the members of the graduating class on his own subject. In addition the law required that every student enter his name with some reputable practising physician for three years as a student in his office—a rather hazy and indefinite relation, for which he paid the physician one hundred dollars a year. If these requirements were met the long-hoped-for sheepskin was forthcoming, and the new M.D. was turned loose on the world.

The combination of simple entry requirements, growing numbers, and a profusion of available medical philosophies guaranteed that a major ailment like tuberculosis would provoke all kinds of theories and attract all kinds of healers, orthodox and eccentric, methodical and mad. Some approaches—arsenic therapy, for example—were destined for the ash heap. Others, like the sanatorium cure, found common cause with what in the twentieth century was fated to become the standard philosophy of medical practice, the contention that the physician's training should be firmly grounded in the basic sciences and in laboratory techniques; that, further, he should approach a patient's illness as if it were a laboratory problem, solving it by a rigorous application of scientific method. But between 1870 and 1910 the situation was fluid, and the budding War on Consumption could hence draw on a variety of competing medical theories, some rigidly experimental, others wildly intuitive, and a highly diverse pool of personnel, from the impeccably rationalistic to the charismatic to the deranged.

Though the sanatorium cure wisely joined the current of modern scientific medicine, adapting itself as the latter grew in force, it is important to remember that its origins were, by modern standards, unscientific. It was, despite the air of authority carried by Brehmer and Dettweiler, a folk cure, rooted in prescientific, even poetic notions of health. Trudeau, though destined for fame as a "Health Hero," was, as he himself would have been the first to admit, not a great scientist. The Adirondack Cottage Sanatorium was a monument to his intuition and his faith, and its survival a monument to his adaptability: as soon as he learned of the startling bacteriological advances of the 1880s he hastened, at no small inconvenience to himself, to master the new laboratory methods. But he was no scientific pioneer, and though it survived into the 1950s, the sanatorium philosophy was a byway, a detour, coexisting amicably with a laboratory-based medicine destined (once antibiotics appeared) to destroy it.

How, if it was such a dinosaur, did the sanatorium flourish for as long as it did? What gap did it fill, left by what failures of the scientist and his laboratory? For the answer, we might go back to March 13, 1877, to a New York City hospital. Let us place the date—eighteen years after the founding of Brehmer's sanatorium at Görbersdorf, five years before the discovery of the tubercle bacillus. Trudeau was then living in obscurity in the Adirondacks, slowly mending, taking on patients, but not yet envisioning a hospital. On that day one Stewart McMurtry, a thirty-two-year-old salesman, was admitted to either Bellevue or Roosevelt Hospital (the records do not show which).

His examining doctor was Francis Delafield, a man destined to be far less famous than Trudeau, but a much better scientist, far more au courant with advanced medical studies. In the late nineteenth century, America was notably weak in the basic sciences, but Delafield bucked the trend. His father, Edward Delafield, had been a pioneer American surgeon and ophthalmologist, founder of the New York Eye and Ear Infirmary; his 1816 dissertation for the College of Physicians and Surgeons was called "An Inaugural Dissertation on Pulmonary Consumption." The younger Delafield took his A.B. at Yale in 1860 and his M.D. at his father's medical school in 1863. He then went to Europe, studied with, and became a disciple of, the renowned German pathologist Rudolf Virchow, a master of painstaking observation and, before the spectacular debut of Robert Koch, perhaps the leading biologist of the nineteenth

century. Delafield, returning to the United States, became a
leading proponent of the scientific method. So much so that in
1886 he was to sponsor a breakaway movement from the
American Medical Association, on the ground that it had become too politicized, an insufficiently learned society. He
wanted "an association in which there will be no medical politics and no medical ethics; . . . We want an association composed of members, each one of whom is able to contribute
something real to the common stock of knowledge and where
he who reads such a contribution feels sure of a discriminating
audience."

It was this exacting figure to whom Stewart McMurtry committed himself for care. According to Delafield's scrupulously
detailed medical history, McMurtry's trouble had begun
fifteen years before with a chronic cough and nasopharyngeal
catarrh. In the view of Delafield, as strict a moralist as he was
a clinician, it was significant as well that McMurtry admitted
to syphilis and a history of intemperance. Six months before his
admission to the hospital he began to feel intermittent pains
in the right side of his chest. These pains worsened until they
began to interfere with his breathing, whereupon they were
joined by chills, sweating, and fever. His appetite slackened
and disappeared. Delafield's chest examination suggested
trouble in McMurtry's right lung. When listened to it sounded
flat; neither voice nor breathing were audible through the
chest wall.

Over the next two weeks, McMurtry worsened steadily. His
pulse continued much faster than normal, and his daily temperature curve traced the undulating pattern of hectic fever,
rising each day toward evening, falling back to normal overnight. As fluid began to accumulate in his chest, breathing
became more difficult. On March 19 Delafield drew eighty-
two ounces of purulent fluid from McMurtry's chest. By March
21 his condition had deteriorated again; he was now vomiting
and delirious. On March 26 Delafield once again aspirated fluid
from his patient, this time extracting twenty-six ounces of pus.
On March 28 McMurtry began sweating profusely; his pulse

faded until it was barely detectable, and at seven in the evening he died.

As was his inveterate and unvarying habit, Delafield conducted an autopsy the next day, carefully studying the condition of McMurtry's lungs, in an effort to correlate it exactly with his symptoms before death. In the right lung Delafield found a cavity three quarters filled with pus. The pleura was thickly coated with fibrin (a product of coagulated blood); air had penetrated into the pleural cavity, normally a partial vacuum. The right lung itself, coated with fibrin and pus, was compressed against the spine, and contained a number of tubercles, some fibrous, some caseous, and some of which had degenerated into cavities.

However sympathetic his bedside manner may have been, Delafield's scrupulously kept notebooks seem slightly chilling in their relentless objectivity, in their preoccupation with charting the course of the disease rather than the relief of the patient's suffering. Yet in so guiding himself, Delafield was simply following the precepts of his mentor Virchow, for whom science was not primarily a search for remedies. That was too hotheaded, too visionary. Rather Virchow saw pathology as the main highway of discovery and viewed the newer branches of scientific medicine (bacteriology, for instance) with suspicion. To him the body was a colony of cells, functioning through a series of complex interactions. Disease was a derangement of these normal relations; the tubercles of consumption were tumors, invaders of lung tissue akin to cancer, a sign of something gone awry in the structural integrity of the lungs. The most promising avenue of investigation for him was therefore the observation of tuberculous tissue's structure rather than the hunt for a microbial cause, and the best medical strategy was to discover, by way of careful postmortem examination, how diseased lungs differed from their healthy counterparts. If one carefully correlated these findings with a full account of the symptoms the patients had evinced before dying, one would, the theory ran, gradually accumulate an accurate and detailed picture of the course of a given disease, and an understanding of how the changes it produced in bodily tissues expressed themselves in symptoms.

It was admirably rigorous, but scarcely suited to raise the physician's stock with a public eager, even desperate, for cures. Small wonder that, however worthy and eminent, Virchow and disciples like Delafield failed to strike a responsive public chord—instead of hope, they offered only a grim account of what had gone fatally wrong. Their interest in restoring health and relieving pain was, though clearly genuine, also secondary. Delafield's scrupulous casebooks suggest a careful and methodical but rather bloodless man, watching spiderlike as his patients struggled in the web of mortal illness, then pouncing, alacritously if not avidly, when they succumbed. He rarely let more than a day go by between a patient's death and the autopsy; often the deceased was on the postmortem table within hours. In his notebook on lung diseases, Delafield recorded fifty-three cases. Many of these patients survived and were discharged, but all of the thirteen people Delafield explicitly identified as consumptive died, most within a few weeks of admission. Implicitly, tuberculosis was hopeless, and Delafield's notes show no interest in any attempt at changing the situation.

Presenting such a bleakly clinical profile to the public, offering, if hope at all, hope only slight and much-deferred, the scientific wing of the medical profession could hardly expect to win much mass allegiance, when every newspaper bore daily advertisements for patent remedies guaranteed to produce cures within a few doses. It required someone with Delafield's near-fanatical devotion to science to pursue it so faithfully in the absence of anything immediate it could do for the comfort or well-being of his patients. But to the physician either concerned with making his patients feel better or with improving the attractiveness, reputation, and wealth of his own threatened profession, or both, such dedication was an unaffordable luxury. Hence the acts of medical bricolage that characterized the closing decades of the nineteenth century; hence Trudeau and the Outdoor Life. To a purist like Delafield it must have seemed like a vital struggle between the pursuit of knowledge and the hunger for money and cheaply won reputation.

Yet it was far more complex. For by the late 1870s both Delafield and his mentor Virchow were proponents of a respectable but already somewhat outdated scientific method. Pathology, without quite falling into disrepute, was being outclassed by a new science, and one that promised immediate, or at least near-term, practical benefits for mankind: bacteriology. The rising figure in this relatively new field, still unknown in America but beginning to be known in Europe and ultimately destined for celebrity, was Robert Koch. Unlike Trudeau he was a scientific experimenter of genius (or at least of indefatigable industry); but unlike Delafield he had a knack for the attention-getting flourish and attracted favorable publicity. His life story came to be as well known in the antituberculosis movement as Trudeau's: in the 1930s the Metropolitan Life Insurance Company circulated a pamphlet biography of him in its Health Heroes series. Koch, born in the Harz Mountains in 1843, survived a childhood that, however unremarkable it may have seemed to a European, very much suited the American palate. It was a struggle with adversity that, thanks to relentless optimism and hard work, turned to triumph. The thirteen little Koch children had, the pamphlet said, much to endure, "surviving mainly on a diet of coarse bread and apples, supplemented twice a week by meat." As a student at Göttingen, the authors approvingly note, Koch "had no love for the usual pastimes of many students at that time, such as fighting and drinking."

Koch began practicing medicine in Silesia, in the neighborhood of Brehmer's fledgling sanatorium, but he was galvanized not by that but rather by the work of Louis Pasteur. While maintaining his country practice, he set himself to determine, if possible, the cause of anthrax, the devastating bacterial infection of cattle and sheep, and sometimes of man. In 1876, after much research, he announced the discovery of the anthrax bacillus at a dramatic meeting at the Botanical Institute in

Breslau. Here as later he displayed an auspicious mixture of dogged industry and dramatic flair. "Drop everything and go at once to Koch!" shouted Julius Cohnheim, an auditor at the Breslau lecture, who, overcome by its revelations, burst in on some colleagues quietly at work in their laboratory. "This man has made a splendid discovery. He has produced something absolutely complete. There is nothing more to be done. I believe Koch will again astonish and shame us with further discoveries."

Such early provincial triumphs soon attracted attention, and Koch moved to Berlin, where, extending his earlier methods, he began, in 1881, a search for the cause of tuberculosis. The gonococcus, the pneumococcus, and the typhus and glanders bacilli had already been discovered, and Koch guessed that a similar organism lay behind tuberculosis. He set for himself a series of criteria that later became known as Koch's Postulates and that remain the standard for identifying the microbial cause of any disease. First, he examined samples of tuberculous tissue and, using various stains, searched for something apparently foreign to the tissue yet consistently found in the presence of the disease. This painstaking process revealed an apparently new bacillus. Then, again through a process of trial and error, elaborating his own earlier experiments, Koch succeeded in separating these bacilli from accompanying but innocent microbes and in growing pure cultures of them. The latter was no easy task, since gelatin, the standard medium for culturing bacteria, didn't work with the tubercle bacillus. Koch's wife pointed out, however, that microbes apparently throve on discarded meat, and this prompted him to try blood serum as a medium, on which, at their normal slow rate, the bacilli finally grew.

The third and most crucial step in the process was to inoculate healthy guinea pigs with the pure bacterial cultures thus obtained in order to see if tuberculosis appeared, and whether, if it did, the suspect bacilli could be found in the lesions of the affected animals. All the guinea pigs Koch inoculated with his cultures were dead within four to six weeks; all showed tubercular lesions in their spleens and livers, from which tubercle bacilli were successfully cultured.

The experiments were concluded within a year and Koch read his resulting paper, "The Aetiology of Tuberculosis," before the Berlin Physiological Society on March 24, 1882. He ended it with a peroration, grandiloquent but merited by the momentous implications of the research:

> Tuberculosis has so far been habitually considered to be a manifestation of social misery, and it has been hoped that an improvement in the latter would reduce the disease. Measures specifically directed against tuberculosis are not known to preventive medicine. But in future the fight against this terrible plague of mankind will deal no longer with an undetermined something but with a tangible parasite, whose living conditions are for the most part known and can be investigated further. The fact that this parasite finds the conditions for its existence only in the animal body and not, as with anthrax bacilli, also outside of it under usual, natural conditions, warrants a particularly favorable outlook for success in the fight against tuberculosis.

The address was met with stunned silence. The methods of the experiment were impeccable, the conclusions unimpeachable. Virchow, by this time the august patriarch of German biological science, sat grim and taciturn among the audience: champion as he was of the claims of pathology, he had for years remained an inveterate enemy to the proposition that consumption was transmissible. But Koch's proof was a devastating blow, not to pathological study but to the idea that the key to diseases and their cure lay in a careful study of the changes they wrought in the affected organs. It seemed only a matter of time until tuberculosis fell before a cure. "No other single physician's work," wrote Allen Krause (a Johns Hopkins physician and frequent contributor to the *American Review of Tuberculosis*) in 1932, "has ever done more to divest mankind of its barbarian habits of thought and action. Such work as his converted incense-burning priests into sure-eyed ministers of health."

But actual events were to prove frustrating. Koch's great talent as a researcher was his patience: tubercle bacilli grow more slowly than do any of the disease-producing organisms discovered before it; he had had to wait nearly three weeks before his medium first showed any sign of culture growth. In 1882 that was unprecedented and might well have provoked a lesser (or less stolid) man to scrap the experiment. But even Koch was unprepared to expect the half century it would in fact take to produce substances capable of retarding the growth of the germ *in vivo*. If scientific medicine was to earn the prestige it craved, results had to be achieved—quickly.

The problem was illustrated by the reception, or rather the nonreception, of Koch's dramatic revelation in practical-minded America, with its disinterest in basic science. In New York the first major public notice of the discovery was a laconic story in the *World* on April 23, nearly a month later:

> Koch has ascertained the exact nature of the parasite which causes consumption. He has propagated it artificially and killed animals with parasites thus produced. Matter expectorated from the lungs of consumptive persons has been found to be swarming with parasites which are highly infective. . . . It is hoped that Koch will develop a harmless form of the tubercular parasite which by inoculation may prevent consumption and thus check a scourge which by Koch's calculation carries off one seventh of the human race.

The *New York Times* ignored the news until May 5, when, in a long editorial, it repeated the information given in the *World* but added a veiled and rather strange attempt to discredit not only Koch but the whole field of bacteriology. The vehicle was an arch story about a fictional Dr. Buhl in Wisconsin, who thought broken legs were caused by a bacterium. "An ardent believer in the germ theory of nearly all disease, [he] claims that he has discovered a vegetable parasite which infests the human trousers, [and] maintains with much plausibility that by inoculating human trousers with this parasite after it has been artificially bred in trousers supplied for the purpose to cattle, men will be fully protected against broken legs." And the American Medical Association, meeting that June in Saint Paul, Minnesota, ignored Koch's discovery entirely, even though the convention began with a ringing paean to science in the keynote address.

In Europe the discovery's warm reception and quickly appreciated significance created their own set of problems. Koch had ended his paper not with an austere recitation of facts but with a peroration envisioning the conquest of tuberculosis. Stunned by his announcement, Europe was breathless with anticipation; but as the years passed, feet began tapping; programs began rustling. Was the new science, so dramatically announced, to fade away without result, returning to the dismal, plodding path laid out by Virchow? Koch felt the pressure acutely and embarked on the search for a cure. He became preoccupied with the subject, even obsessed—publicity kindled the expectation for further spectacular results, and the very support he had been receiving from the Prussian government turned into quiet, implicit pressure. And in fact the whole European medical fraternity was expecting something. Bacteriology had decisively wrested the palm from pathology in disclosing the cause of a dread disease; now the world was waiting expectantly for the cure.

Koch, loath to disappoint, allowed his ambition to outrun his judgment. In the late fall of 1890 (while Trudeau was laboring in the Adirondacks to build his hospital from a single crude cottage, husbanding his first few patients through the rigors of the Adirondack winter) he announced a cure at a meeting of the International Medical Congress in Berlin. After years of rumors, the reaction was explosive; nothing like the delayed and grudging response that, at least in the United States, had met the 1882 announcement. Koch's address was translated almost at once into various languages; the news merited large headlines in major newspapers; pamphlets appeared explaining the new cure and praising Koch lavishly.

Koch himself began his presentation with an unusual and, to the soberer elements of the scientific community, disquieting announcement. He would, he said, discuss neither the preparation nor the composition of the remedy, volunteering only the information that it was "a clear, brownish liquid, which keeps its strength without any special precautions being taken." He went on to explain that the drug was to be administered by injection in the back, either between the shoulder blades or in the lumbar region. With a sense of drama honed by his track record of stunning announcements, he then revealed that he had tested the remedy first by administering it to himself:

> Three or four hours after the injection I felt pains in the limbs, fatigue, inclination to cough, difficulty in breathing, all which speedily increased; in the fifth hour I was seized with an unusually violent fit of shivering, which lasted nearly an hour; at the same time there was sickness, vomiting, and the temperature of the body rose to 39.6°; after about twelve hours all these symptoms gradually grew less, the temperature fell, and by the next day was again normal.

In healthy individuals Koch observed that a small injection of the "lymph," as it came to be called, provoked little or no reaction; but in the tubercular, the same dosage produced a violent feverish attack lasting from twelve to fifteen hours. This attack was followed by a local reaction on which Koch based his claim that the lymph was a cure. Any visible tubercular lesions (such as facial spots in tubercular lupus, or tuberculous infections of the glands, bones, or joints) began to swell, turn red, and grow painful. Lupus spots then turned brown and became necrotic, and, as the fever of the general reaction subsided, they began to shrink and eventually disappeared. In patients with pulmonary consumption, Koch asserted, the injection was followed at first by increased coughing and expectoration; he inferred that what went on with the lupus sores was also happening invisibly with the tubercles in the lungs—a brief flare-up in activity followed by the destruction of the diseased tissue. He reported that in the majority of tested patients the cough and spitting gradually lessened after the initial eruption; in the most successful cases they vanished entirely.

Considering the maelstrom into which his discovery was to plunge him, it is worth pointing out that Koch himself carefully limited his claims. He noted that the lymph's apparent effect was to provoke the body's chemistry into an attack on the sites of infection, and though the inference was that the tubercle bacilli would perish in the resulting conflagration, they were not apparently the goal of direct attack, and hence might escape. "It will be quite possible in apparently cured cases of tuberculosis of the lungs or joints to determine whether the process of disease is really terminated, or whether there may not still be some few diseased spots which might cause the disease to break out afresh, spreading its ravages like sparks from under smouldering ashes."

The reaction to this address was thunderous; all the claims struck the public imagination; none of the reservations did. An avalanche of the ill and desperate descended on Berlin. Lodging became nearly impossible to obtain. The English *Review of Reviews* published a cartoon, "Koch as the New St. George," slaying the tubercle bacillus. Sensational and heartrending stories made their way into the popular press—consumptives dying on the very trains that brought them to the city of their last hope. The tubercular son of a rich Berlin merchant, curing at Menton, decided impulsively to return home. In the excitement, his younger sister died of a sudden heart attack, and witnessing this her brother suffered a fatal hemorrhage. In the office handling Koch's correspondence, Sir Arthur Conan Doyle, reporting on the furor that followed the announcement of the cure, noted on the floor a pile of letters four feet across and high as a man's knee, all demanding the miraculous lymph.

Professional reactions were, by contrast, much more ambivalent, even turbulent. Orthodox scientists were outraged by Koch's refusal to divulge the composition of the lymph. It could not be analyzed or subjected to informed scrutiny; such secretiveness in the pillar of contemporary scientific medicine was thought particularly scandalous. Conservative scientific publications excoriated the erstwhile hero for blocking the flow of scientific information and violating the code of openness the profession had been upholding against the secrecy of the quacks, medical sectarians, and concocters of patent medicines.

At first such cavils did little to quell the rising excitement: through December of 1890 Koch treated between seven hundred and eight hundred patients. But hopes, fanned high, rapidly began to weaken. The patients died at or above rates that would be anticipated for untreated consumptives. Whatever its potential merits as a diagnostic tool (the difference in reaction between the uninfected and the infected was sharp and unmistakable), it was, it soon fell out, no cure. By 1891, 2,172 consumptives had been treated at Berlin hospitals with 17,500 injections of the lymph. Of 1,061 patients with internal manifestations of the disease, 13 were reported cured, 171 much improved, and 194 slightly improved. But 586 were no better and 46 had died.

Rudolf Virchow, now sixty-nine, and perhaps remembering the humiliation of having to sit dumbfounded through Koch's 1882 triumph, strode purposefully into the autopsy room. He performed postmortems on twenty-one patients who had died after treatment with the lymph, reaching two conclusions that amounted to a rearguard triumph for pathology over the upstart work of the bacteriologists. First, though the Koch fluid did often provoke a reaction that in turn destroyed tuberculous tissue, it did not in any way affect the bacilli, and in many cases the treatment left active sites of infection on which, apparently, the reaction had no effect. Second, in very weak patients, the broken-down disease tissue, instead of being expectorated or otherwise eliminated from the body, remained in the lungs, perhaps serving as a source for the further catastrophic spread of the disease.

Pressured by the failure of his remedy, Koch retreated. In January 1891 he revealed its composition: "a glycerine extract derived from the pure cultivation of tubercle bacilli." He was unable, he now admitted, to hazard more than a guess as to the identity of the active component, speculating only that it was perhaps a toxin released by the microbe. Harmful to the tissues surrounding the sites of infection, he guessed, it eventually destroyed them, and in so doing deprived the still-active bacilli of their natural medium. This humiliating debacle was more than an embarrassment for Koch; it was a setback for the reputation of medicine, particularly in the United States, where doctors were trying to improve their hitherto uncertain lot.

The shame became particularly acute when, in the aftermath of the lymph's failure, a rather seamy tale emerged. On November 29, 1890, Dr. Gustav von Gossler, the Prussian Minister of Worship and Public Instruction, spoke before the Prussian Diet and tried to explain to the members' satisfaction why the government had discouraged Koch from making his formula public. First, the minister explained, they wanted to prevent it from getting into "the hands of swindlers." Then von Gossler further revealed that they "had come to an agreement with Dr. Koch that the remedy should be produced under the management of the state." He added, rather implausibly, that "even if it was not possible to produce the quantity necessary, yet the whole world would be glad to hear Prussia had put her stamp on it."

By the spring of 1891 it had emerged that in fact the Prussian government meant to sell the lymph for profit and, more shocking yet, to divide the profits with Koch. The government's high-toned pronouncement, and Koch's initial assertion that he was withholding the formula only because "my work is not yet completed," began to throw off the stench of cynicism. As the *British Medical Journal* put it, such revelations were "of a somewhat disquieting character. It has been said . . . Dr. Koch and each of his assistants had accepted a large immediate payment, and that they were to receive a royalty upon all sales in the future." The *Journal* then noted disapprovingly that, "the arrangement, it must be admitted, would partake far too much of the commercial transaction to be agreeable to the traditions of the medical profession, or the customs of men of science."

In the United States, more hospitable to the spirit of enterprise, Koch was treated more gently: the *Journal of the American Medical Association* strained to avoid condemning Koch directly; but the situation was agonizing, all the more so as evidence accumulated that the remedy was in fact entirely ineffective and often detrimental. A Chicago physician, E. Fletcher Ingals, writing in the February 21, 1891, issue of the *Journal*, quoted a letter from a friend on the scene in Berlin.

> Dr. Koch's remedy is still with us, but becoming less popular daily, if I may judge from students and others who have an opportunity of witnessing the treatment. Beside the French and not a few German opponents who are animated by feelings of rivalry or the like, some there are of late who, closely observing the matter, do not hesitate to condemn the treatment as both fruitless, dangerous, and unscientific, since it seems to diminish the patient's strength and physical resistance by its local and general powerful action, and hence a condition favorable to the extension of tuberculosis. . . . A friend of mine, candid and intelligent, who is taking a private course in physical diagnosis under one of Gerhardt's assistants, and seeing much of the cases, gives very unfavorable reports.

Generally, the *Journal of the American Medical Association* treated Koch with deference; it was not eager to drag a heaven-sent hero through the mire in retribution for one failed experiment and a few lapses of judgment. And in spite of the failure of the Koch lymph in such spectacular circumstances, such was his hold on the profession that it took years for its allure to fade. Trudeau, for example, though one of the first to realize the substance was far from a cure, continued to experiment with it until his death in 1915; a number of his patients were given courses of it.

In tuberculosis, at least, the patient, methodical observation

167

of pathology had given way to the spectacular successes of bacteriology. Their victory was pyrrhic, but the followers of Virchow gloated over its first, and glaringly publicized, debacle. "Twenty years ago," one such physician wrote in *Aesclepiad*, "we were steering well and steadily towards great principles on the preventive as well as on the curative side of medicine. Then there crept in the wild enthusiasm of bacteriological research, . . . a positive insanity when accepted as the one absorbing pursuit, . . . leading to Babel with its confusion of tongues, and separating, for a time, our modern art of cure from the accumulated treasures of knowledge, wisdom and light of over one thousand years." And, indeed, pathology had not been stopped in its tracks: in 1890 Delafield was still at work in the dissecting rooms at Roosevelt and Bellevue hospitals. The last recorded case of tuberculosis in his notebook was a patient named Guiseppe [*sic*] Arnoldi, admitted on September 28, 1890, in the midst of the frenzy in Berlin. Delafield tracked his condition diligently through bouts of dyspnea, weight loss, weakness, and a final catastrophic buildup of fluid in his lungs. He died on December 11 at nine-thirty in the morning. At three-fifteen that afternoon Delafield began the autopsy.

The crisis in the War on Consumption, in other words, coincided with a crisis in the medical profession, particularly in the United States. How was medicine to define itself, how was it to validate its claim to authority and public trust? The conquest of tuberculosis was a tempting answer; if the world's leading cause of death could be controlled by the forces of orthodox medicine, its worthiness could no longer stand in doubt. The events of 1882 seemed to assure that this goal could best be reached through the bacteriological laboratory, whose methods doctors quickly hastened to embrace. But now, in 1890, the whole fragile enterprise was shaken, and to a skeptical observer it must have indeed looked as if the doctors were laboring amidst the ruins of Babel. Brehmer, Dettweiler, Trudeau, and their followers, however sympathetic to science, were heirs to a more informal tradition. But they could point to concrete results, while the scientists, claiming a closer grip on truth, were at war among themselves. And divided though they were, they all, pathologists and bacteriologists alike, had to face competition from outside the medical fraternity—faith healers, galvanologists (who ran electric currents through their patients), and patent-medicine hucksters.

The result of this impasse was improvisation. *Ex post facto* the road from the discovery of 1882 to the emergence of antibiotics in the 1940s looks long but relatively straight. It wasn't; it was forked. On the one hand, the scientific researchers marched forward, encouraged by their progress, but finding the cure for consumption elusive. On the other, the sanatorium movement proceeded, eclectically absorbing whatever seemed promising or useful—science, psychology, social theory, popular philosophy, free enterprise, the schemes of philanthropy. As medicine glued itself more and more firmly to science, the antituberculosis movement followed, but nonetheless retained its attachment to a system of ideas not strictly, and sometimes not at all, scientific. It thus blossomed against the long-term current of the profession, but was also doomed to vanish with the ultimate triumph of science.

For by the 1890s a number of leading physicians had concluded that the only way to discipline the chaos of contemporary medicine was to limit the number of practitioners and to standardize what they studied. And what they studied, the consensus went, should not be homeopathy, optimism, Thomsonianism, or any other mythical system, but hard science. They agitated to link the nation's major medical schools firmly to the rigor and the prestige of science and to close down the marginal ones. Their advocacy reached a critical point with Abraham Flexner's 1910 report to the Carnegie Foundation, *Medical Education in the United States and Canada.* This report was essentially the crucible in which modern medicine was compounded: brief, firm, unclouded by doubts or pusillanimous reservations, it focused sharply a number of ideas that had hitherto circulated through the profession but remained diffuse.

169

For Flexner, the linchpin of medical education was the mastery of the experimental method. What could be clearer? Medicine was science; hence the doctor's training should approximate the scientist's as closely as possible (although nowhere in his report does he take seriously, or even address, the idea that medical practice is an art, operating as much by intuition as induction). Earlier nineteenth-century scientists like Virchow were much preoccupied with the accurate description of phenomena; the rage for experiment emerged during the latter quarter of the century, and it was this, rather than the earlier method, that Flexner enjoined on the medical school of the future. To him, the physician was faced, day by day, with problems. These were to be assessed by careful observation; a hypothesis was to be formed about their cause, and that hypothesis tested. The physician, he wrote, "is confronted by a definite situation. . . . He must needs seize its details, and only powers of observation trained in actual experimentation will enable him to do so. The patient's history, conditions, symptoms, form his data. Thereupon he, too, frames his working hypothesis, now called a diagnosis." True, illness sometimes eludes forthright analysis; the living human can't be confined to the pure atmosphere of the laboratory—his existence merges on many frontiers and with untrackable complexity into the world of which he is part. But this, for Flexner, didn't compromise the general validity of the method, and he dismissed any such reservations lightly: "in the twilight region probabilities are substituted for certainties."

One can see how revolutionary, also how less than inevitable, the model Flexner offered to the profession was, especially when contrasted with the methods of the practitioners examined so far. Koch was the very model for Flexner's physician of the future—sober experimenter, driven by the need to relieve suffering, but controlled by an equally acute passion for certainty. Every postulate demanded corroboration by evidence: search the diseased tissue for the pathogenic organism, culture that organism under carefully supervised conditions. Reintroduce the animalcules thus cultured into test animals and ascertain that in every case the disease occurs. Then, to be absolutely sure, excise diseased tissue from the infected animals: in every case the suspected pathogen must be recovered.

Then there was Delafield, the representative of an earlier school, impeccably scientific, but cast in a different mold. Where Koch worked in the laboratory, Delafield labored in the hospital; Koch solved mysteries, Delafield described them. Nowhere in his notebook does he show an immediate interest in the cause of consumption—he was obsessed instead with what it did to the structure of the lungs it afflicted. And if on the one hand that made him seem cold-bloodedly detached from suffering, passively willing to explore without intervening, it might also be argued on his behalf that he was less arrogant than Koch, who in his laboratory was meddling in the natural course of cause and effect—isolating a chunk of nature and guiding its fate as if he were a demiurge. The bacteriologist, the new scientist, the model Flexner chose for the physician, was not merely content to observe, not even to palliate: he would instead play with the units of disease as if they were chips in a game—pluck the pathogens from the sufferer, propagate them in a universe he himself creates, watch them grow, inflict them on an experimental animal, and recover them again like a farmer corralling sheep from their pasture.

In the 1870s, at least, Trudeau represented a second alternative to the experimental model: folklore. The pioneers of the sanatorium movement in its earliest years—Brehmer, Dettweiler, Trudeau—were relying neither on the careful observation of consumption's clinical course nor on anything like controlled experiment. They were merely doing what came naturally, improvising, relying on intuition and afflatus, absorbing generally current cultural ideas about health (medical and nonmedical) and transforming them into a regimen of life. The Bavarians who exercised in Brehmer's Silesian retreat (on the false theory that a sluggish heart caused the illness), the Frankfurt burghers who rested at Dettweiler's (on the possibly true idea that inactivity cured it), the factory girls who rested

and exercised at Trudeau's (on the characteristically pragmatic premise that both had merit)—all were active participants in the cure. None were mere passive subjects of observation or distant prospects from the vantage point of the
laboratory. Their doctors were intent, to the best of their abili-
ties, on helping them, theory and method be hanged. None
were associated with the fringe of Victorian medicine, with its
sects or its crazes—none dosed the patients, for example, with
arsenic, a much-touted mid-century remedy that its enthusiasts claimed as a sure cure for consumption. But still,
before the identification of the microscopic enemy, these doctors were not content with the patient scholarship of a Virchow or a Delafield. They wanted results, and could plausibly
claim them.

Why, then, apart from the power of fashion, should it have
been the ways of Koch that were destined to dominate the
development of modern medicine? If they had fostered a triumph in 1882, they had also spawned a disaster in 1891, at the
same time that Trudeau and his colleagues in the anticonsumption movement could credibly claim cures and could
point by way of corroboration to a falling death rate from
tuberculosis. The simple answer is perhaps supplied by
Flexner himself. It is only deep in the body of his report that
he advocates scientific method as the basis of medicine. At the
outset he is far more concerned to denounce the proliferation
of doctors and to call for a cutback. "The improvement of
medical education," he announces in his first chapter, "cannot
. . . be resisted on the ground that it will destroy schools and
restrict output: that is precisely what is needed. . . . The country needs fewer and better doctors." Recording that one of the
more desperate proprietary medical schools had, in an advertisement, offered prospective students a free European trip if
they attended, he argues that the country had clearly produced too many doctors with indifferent skills; the output of
new physicians should not be allowed to proliferate on the
ground either that it offered the public a wider choice or that
it opened the profession to the poor:

The medical profession is a social organ, created not for the purpose of gratifying the inclinations or preferences of certain individuals, but as a means of promoting health, physical vigor, happiness. . . . Your "poor boy" has no right, natural, indefeasible, or acquired, to enter upon the practice of medicine unless it is best for society that he should.

Flexner's heat here is perhaps revealing. On the one hand he posits the energetic (but unsubstantiated) claim that medicine would improve if fewer were called to it; then he offers the still more energetic (and superfluous) assertion that the "poor boy" had no God-given right to enter the profession. The implicit reasoning—though Flexner might well deny it—is that the envisioned fewer doctors would be better because they were gentlemen. The obvious argument, that restricting access to medical schools would confine them to the most talented applicants, is never explicitly made.

As Flexner envisioned it, the chief function of enthroning science as the standard for medical education is that, being expensive, laborious, and demanding of personal attention by instructor to student, it must necessarily be offered to fewer students.

With the advent of the laboratory, in which every student possesses a locker where his individual microscopes, reagents, and other paraphernalia are stored for his personal use; with the advent of the small group bedside clinic, in which every student is responsible for a patient's history and for a trial diagnosis, suggested, confirmed, or modified by his own microscopial and chemical examination of blood, urine, sputum, and other tissues, the privileges of the medical school can no longer be open to casual strollers from the highway.

No longer is rote memory of lecture notes to be the lingua franca of the medical school; the student is to prepare for his clinical instruction by obtaining a thorough background in chemistry, biology, and physics on a college level.

173

It cannot have escaped Flexner, and plainly did not escape the leaders of the medical profession at the time, that whatever improvement this proposed reform might render in the quality of the average American doctor over time, it would radically reduce supply against a constant demand: the physician who survived the Flexnerian triage would find himself in an enviable economic position. Though it was never fully implemented, Flexner's plan called for only twenty-seven medical schools throughout the country. New York, the most populous state, was to be furnished with only two—one in New York City, one in Buffalo.

And along with economic power would come the sine qua non that modern analysts of both medicine and professionalism in general have identified as the essence of a profession as against more menial kinds of work—a control over the conditions of work by the worker himself, independent of external authority. In fact a concordat of sorts emerged over time between the physicians and governmental authorities that might have controlled them, allowing them fundamental independence. This in turn allowed them to purvey to the public what one observer, Magali Sarfatti Larson, has identified as a peculiarly numinous product: an aura of professional skill. Certainly, as the nineteenth century drew to a close the public had more and more money to spend on anything they thought worth the purchasing. And as medicine grew more and more respectable, it could charge more for its wares. Yet the commodity being offered was invisible; was even, as Larson calls it, fictitious: a claim to esoteric knowledge that was, in practice, rarely visible to the purchaser and that, real or supposed, might or might not have bearing on the treatment the patient actually got.

So the problem, for the founders of modern medicine, was to persuade the public (and themselves) that they were masters of a specialized and hard-to-acquire knowledge worth paying for, and likely to yield results. Yet, as Larson also remarks, a group bent on thoroughly sequestering its work from public control, yet eager to persuade the same public of its value,

faces a problem. On the one hand its skills need to be demon-
strably real, open to scrutiny and approval. Yet unless they're
sufficiently arcane, anyone might learn them, and the claim to
a need for exclusivity vanishes. So for all its intimidating raz-
zle-dazzle, the experimental method and the flowering of
elaborate technology that followed from it are dangerous ac-
quisitions for doctors, precisely because, being mechanically
repeatable, they are tasks anyone might learn.

But a profession also gains some of its prestige from the fact
that, though surrounded by a reassuringly certain network of
scientific rules, the center of its work is indeterminate—we
ascribe much of the doctor's virtue not to his mastery of quanti-
tative techniques alone but to a fund of judgment and un-
defined skill that has sprung up in him as a consequence of his
scientific training. Ultimately, one is willing to submit to the
judgment of one's physician because one credits him with the
mastery of "means that escape rules and . . . are attributed to
the virtualities of the producers." Practitioners, asked to describe the nature of their work, consistently emphasize the
indeterminacy of it, the frequency of their reliance on inspiration rather than upon the application of clear scientific laws,
and hence, success or failure in treatment is attributed not to
chance or the inevitable workings of nature but to the virtue
or the inadequacy of the doctor. Or, as Eliot Freidson, perhaps
the leading modern historian of medical professionalism, has
said, "like political or economic power, professional authority
teeters between glory and ruin and is prone to claim its glory
more because of its risk of ruin than because of its accomplishment."

There is, in other words, a paradox in the way modern medicine constituted itself. It based its educational system, and the
consequent economically enriching shrinkage in the number
of available doctors, on the proposition that medical education
had to be conducted strictly according to the principles of
experimental science. Yet in actual medical practice the individual doctor and his patient have both come to ascribe his
professional virtue not to the certainties of science but to vir-

tue in the most primitive sense of that word—an almost mystical power, general rather than specific, conferred on him by his scientific training but not directly attributable to it.

As modern medicine has developed, it is arguable that this latent conflict has never been resolved; that it remains as the source of much ambivalence about medicine, both within the profession and outside. We expect our doctors to be men of science, offering answers as clear, and results as concrete, as those produced from controlled experiments. Yet we also expect them to be shamans, possessors of the power to soothe and ameliorate, drawing from sources deeper and more magical than those scientists can tap. The modern hospital is a schizophrenic temple—it bristles with technology and equipment and is prodigiously organized; a policy, usually written, governs every possibility. And the more dramatic the suffering, the more equipment arrives, the more method descends, as if to swamp the clamors of pain and death. They can be drowned out if they can't be prevented. At the same time we demand comfort of physicians, want them to be well versed in personal skills, and expect of them healing virtues we'd call magic if we weren't conditioned to think of them as scientific.

The antituberculosis movement managed, in part, to reconcile these contradictions. The sanatorium was a hospital, but it was also a hometown with social amenities and a relation between patient and healer that went beyond the technical and approached the familial. In part it ran on orthodox scientific lines, keeping up with advances in treatment through a network of journals and professional societies. But it also tapped other resources; it was a folk phenomenon, part summer camp continued through the winter, part college, part rural agrarian utopia, part family, benevolently guided by a paterfamilias in the medical director. It achieved a brief marriage between two opposed philosophies of healing, one rationalistic, the other intuitive, one elitist, the other populist. The cohabitation came to an end with antibiotics, but it pointed out a direction medicine might have taken, yet in the end did not.

Yet while it continued, the War on Consumption inevitably

attracted, thanks to its eclecticism, distinct and not always entirely harmonious groups. Not only physicians but social reformers of all stripes, businessmen, community activists, and clergy; all happily gathered under the banner. They might, of course, have gathered their energies around other frightful Victorian plagues, like cholera or diphtheria. But tuberculosis was more frequent, more fatal, and, more important, longer-lived. The other diseases—yellow fever or cholera—tended to sweep through the cities in horrendous but short-term waves; consequently they could not have supported a major crusade, sustained over years and supported by a large-scale establishment. A bureaucracy, an empire, a dynasty might be built on tuberculosis; the others could sustain only a campaign, dying as the brief epidemic wave ebbed.

This was manifest in the first significant agitation for a War on Consumption, initiated in New York City by Hermann Biggs in 1889 and again in 1893. In a report to the city health department, Biggs recommended that hospitals segregate tuberculosis patients, that free tuberculosis hospitals be established, and that the city form a corps of health officers charged with tracking individual cases. Biggs enlisted the press, drummed up public support, and was quickly followed by Lawrence F. Flick of Philadelphia, who founded an antituberculosis society there in 1892. Over the next decade the movement grew steadily and fast. Though Biggs and Flick were both physicians, their movement attracted only lukewarm enthusiasm from the profession as a whole, and as a result they enlisted the participation of laypeople, who became increasingly important. A pattern of cooperation between the profession and community leaders thus set in and became a hallmark of the movement. As C. E. A. Winslow, a leading historian of public health, remarked, "the discovery of the possibilities of wide-spread social organization as a means of controlling disease was one which may almost be placed alongside the discovery of the germ theory of disease itself as a factor in the evolution of the modern public health campaign."

But between 1900 and 1902 the earliest attempts to set up

a national tuberculosis association, led by Clark Bell (president of the Medico-Legal Society of New York and a layman), ran into trouble because of jockeying for power between physicians and laymen. For a time in 1903 the fraternity contemplated fratricide: there were briefly two rival congresses, one controlled by Bell and centered in New York, the other by the physicians Daniel Lewis and George Brown and headquartered in Atlanta.

An impending imbroglio was resolved when the leading tuberculosis lights gathered at an exhibit in Baltimore in 1904, sponsored by the Maryland Commission on Tuberculosis. Trudeau, S. Adolphus Knopf, Vincent Bowditch (son of Henry and founder of the first Massachusetts sanatorium at Sharon), and Flick all came. So did perhaps the most influential medical figures of the time, Sir William Osler and William Welch, author of a standard medical textbook. Thus though the goal was reconciliation, the peace conference was dominated by an intimidating show of medical prestige. Nonetheless, in the end the newly formed association resolved to encourage participation by all interested parties. It aimed to sponsor scientific research, but also declared an equal interest in agitating for appropriate legislation, educating the public, and offering relief to the victims of consumption. Trudeau appears to have functioned at the conference more as a tutelary deity than an active agitant (he was in poor health), but his eclectic and unexclusive spirit won the day. The cooperative model of the sanatorium was thus extended to the movement at large. In later years there would be tension and disagreement, but the principle of collective effort remained alive.

True, the physicians would ultimately triumph. But in the meanwhile the campaign attracted others, a diverse lot less likely to be thought of as participants in a medical enterprise. For this was a crusade in its power to transcend social barriers as well as in its attack on a common enemy.

7

"Plainly Designed for the Public Good":
Reform, Philanthropy, and Business

We are prepared, when necessary, to introduce and
enforce, and the people are ready to accept, measures
which might seem radical and arbitrary, if they were not
plainly designed for the public good, and evidently
beneficent in their effects. Even among the most ignorant
of our foreign-born population, few or no indications of
resentment are exhibited to the exercise of arbitrary
powers in sanitary matters.

—HERMANN BIGGS, ADDRESSING
THE BRITISH MEDICAL ASSOCIATION,
MONTREAL, SEPTEMBER 3, 1897

One night in 1903 Ernest Poole entered a choked room in a
rear tenement at 18 Clinton Street on the Lower East Side.
The object of his visit was a young Rumanian Jew, in the last
stages of consumption, who lay on the floor of the ten-foot-
square room, gasping for breath: *"Luft—luft—gib mir luft*
[Breath—breath—give me breath]."

Poole, a member of the Charity Organization Society of the
City of New York's antituberculosis committee, was shocked
by the desperation of the sufferer, but even more shocked by
the squalor of his surroundings and the knowledge that they
were endlessly duplicated in neighboring blocks.

With every breath I felt the heavy, foul odor from poverty, ignorance, filth, disease. In this room ten feet square
six people lay on the floor packed close, rubbing the heavy
sleep from tired eyes, and staring at us dumbly. Two small
windows gave them air, from a noisome court—a pit
twenty feet across and five floors deep. The other room
was only a closet six feet by seven, with a grated window
high up opening on an air shaft eighteen inches wide. And

in that closet, four more were sleeping, three on a bed, one in a cradle.

Even in 1903, after more than a decade of tenement reform in New York, there were some 361,000 such rooms in the city, forcing beds of misery, crime, and epidemic disease. Ever since the mid-nineteenth century, social reformers had been agonizing over the city's growing and apparently intractable slums; even to the halting science of the time it was evident that their filth and crowding spawned bouts of infectious disease like cholera, typhus, and diphtheria, apart from all the social ills they bred. But with the discovery that tuberculosis was transmissible and, in conditions of darkness, crowding, and poor nutrition contagious, the slums took on a new, more sinister air. Typhus and cholera might arouse panic, but (with notable exceptions) they confined themselves largely to brief but deadly upsurges in the poverty-stricken districts in which they originated. But consumption carried off millions, spreading without the apocalyptic warning signals given by other diseases. And it was omnipresent, never fading away, either from the population or its consciousness. With Koch's discovery, in other words, the slums cast a new and terrifying shadow on the comfortable neighborhoods surrounding them.

The fledgling antituberculosis movement was quick to seize on the image of the tenement as an embodiment of the threat of consumption; the tenement reform movement was quick to seize on tuberculosis as an added reason to clear the slums. Both had their roots in the sanitary reform movement, which had begun in the United States as early as the 1840s. But because of worsening conditions in the cities, a more effective industry able to publicize them, and the emergence of a few pioneering individuals, like Jacob Riis, Trudeau, and Ernest Poole, who were able to translate theories and good wishes into potent images consumable by the general public, the reform movement gained strong momentum in the 1880s and 1890s. Thus it would be reductive to consider the antituberculosis movement largely as a medical phenomenon that created around itself a whole subculture, centering on the sanatorium and drawing its ethos eclectically from many sources, ranging from science to utopian idealism to a sentimental vision of the American rural past. Relatively few of the victims of consumption ever spent time in a sanatorium: most were either too poor to afford it or unwilling to undergo the confinement and regimentation of the cure. The crusaders therefore had to conduct their campaign not only in the sanatoriums, not only in the printed media, but also in the cities. The homebound tubercular had to be treated; the spread of the disease had to be controlled; the conditions that encouraged it had to be wiped out. This campaign had as its battleground not a controlled community but the whole nation, particularly its cities. And its weapons were not rules and daily routines to which hopeful patients eagerly subscribed themselves, but laws, the gross implements of social control. Much of the War on Tuberculosis was a political struggle; Tammany Hall was as important in its history as were the Adirondacks and the Rockies. It was a campaign that involved government and business; its battleground was the city.

Physically the nineteenth-century city was a more complex place in some ways than it is now. New York was typical in this respect; its gridlike thoroughfares were only the superficial channels of its activity. The population, particularly the poor, lived in a warren of courts, alleyways, galleries, and tunnels behind the streets. To a modern eye, the latter look small in scale, quaint, almost rural: photographs of Mulberry Bend, in the 1880s the city's most notorious slum district, show a rather pleasing perspective of two-story brick and clapboard houses, sociable, even intimate in scale. It was behind these streetscapes that the hells began. As the crush of immigrant population descended on the city, landlords built ramshackle structures, called back tenements, in the open yards behind their original buildings. They were thrown up in every available nook and cranny, often at odd angles, were built as high as cheap construction would permit, and were connected to the street by networks of improvised alleys. These rear tenements were the worst accommodations in the city, dark, cramped, often without adequate water or sewage. Their very complexity, their darkness, their mystery, made them potent images of disease as well as hotbeds of it. As the mysterious workings of illness had to be investigated, and their depredations on the body repaired, so the dark, entangled courtyards and alleys had to be explored, then cleared up. The two projects were allied in their imagery, and they were allied in fact; the slum clearers and the health reformers took common cause.

Jacob Riis was the most effective of the tenement-house reformers. Others had anticipated him, but nothing galvanized the public as did the 1890 publication of *How the Other Half Lives,* a grim and heavily dramatized but not sensationalized portrait of life in New York's tenement districts. Perhaps the book's decisive power lay in its illustrations, copied from Riis's own photography, which plunged him into the abyss of tenement life to the extent that during one foray into a lodging house he actually set the place on fire with his flash apparatus. His text is alternately affecting and shocking, since it combines an acute rendering of the miseries of poverty with an unpredictable bigotry toward some of those who suffer it; at times Riis's outrage over dreadful conditions becomes inseparable from his contempt for the hapless ignorance of the victims. He is notably anti-Semitic, for example, flailing at Jews for the very initiative and enterprise he elsewhere touts, blaming them for the very industriousness he himself realizes will eventually lift them out of poverty. He is also harsh toward the Italians (misliking their raucous street life), the Irish, and the Chinese, reserving praise only for the Germans and the Bohemians.

Whatever the defects in his ethnic sympathies, Riis's evocation of slum life was vivid, and his impressions coalesced with those of the antituberculosis movement, for the central image of *How the Other Half Lives* is suffocation, darkness, claustrophobia, the ubiquitousness of poisonous air, awful smells, and the closing in of walls and inmates.

Bottle Alley . . . is a fair specimen of its kind, wherever found. Look into any of these houses, everywhere the same piles of rags, of malodorous bones and musty paper [are found]. Here is a "flat" of "parlor" and two pitch-dark coops called bedrooms. Truly, the bed is all there is room for. The family tea-kettle is on the stove, doing duty for the time being as a wash-boiler. By night it will have returned to its proper use again, a practical illustration of how poverty in "the Bend" makes both ends meet. One, two, three beds are there, if the old boxes and heaps of foul straw can be called by that name; a broken stove with crazy pipe from which smoke leaks at every joint, a table of rough boards propped up on boxes, piles of rubbish in the corner. The closeness and smell are appalling. How many people sleep here?

Attempts to promulgate health standards had been made as early as the 1860s, and by 1890 there were laws on the books, at least in New York. Builders were made subject to a code setting minimum ventilation and fenestration for each room. But a combination of indifference, political corruption, the inventiveness of landlords, and the sheer press of the city's increasing population had effectively nullified whatever reforms had been undertaken. In the 1890s the situation had come to be felt desperate, and the knowledge that the White Plague was spreading through these blighted neighborhoods added to the urgency.

Riis's example stimulated a number of anticonsumption crusaders, who described the slums similarly but as particular seedbeds of tuberculosis. Perhaps the most notable of these writers was Poole, who began a long career as a muckraker in 1903 with *The Plague in Its Stronghold,* a tract included as part of a report on tuberculosis by the Charity Organization Society and afterward issued separately as a pamphlet. After his opening description of 18 Clinton Street, Poole conjures up the special horrors of tuberculosis. Its new late-nineteenth-century nickname, the White Plague, was the product of a conscious propaganda campaign, designed to link it in the public imagination with the more familiar and apocalyptic

plagues, to rouse for its slow and unobtrusive spread the same
sort of terror typhus and bubonic plague once provoked.

Poole himself appreciates the paradox that mankind's most
destructive disease had somehow never called up a fear pro-
portionate to its seriousness:

> It is a Plague in disguise. Its ravages are insidious, slow.
> They have never yet roused people to a great, sweeping
> action. The Black Plague in London is ever remembered
> with horror. It lived one year; it killed fifty thousand. The
> Plague Consumption kills this year in Europe over a mil-
> lion; and this has been going on not for one year but for
> centuries. It is the Plague of all plagues—both in age and
> in power—insidious, steady, unceasing.

In Poole's pamphlet the New York stronghold of the Plague
was the city's tenement population; but, astute propagandist
that he was, he felt the need for a more specific focus. Hence
the "Lung Block." Poole estimated there were at least twenty
thousand cases of tuberculosis in New York, primarily in the
slum districts. But the block bounded by Cherry, Catherine,
Hamilton, and Market streets was infamous, even allowing for
its neighborhood. At the time, New York's population aver-
aged 478 per acre, but 4,000 humans were packed into the
Lung Block, which had, over the course of nine years, 265
reported cases of consumption (many more, Poole assumed,
went unreported, since residents were born, arrived, disappeared, and died without ever appearing in any official record). Houses, either fronting the streets or crammed into the
stinking yards behind, went by evocative names rather than by
numbers—the Ink Pot, the Bucket, the Barracks, the Morgue.

Poole was a more acute, perhaps because a more clinical,
observer of the oppressive atmosphere of the Lung Block than
even Riis was of the Mulberry Bend neighborhood a few blocks
to the northwest. He photographed one tenement house, six
stories high, its inner rooms ventilated only by a minelike shaft
six feet long and twelve inches wide. The aptly named Bucket
opened on a dank courtyard:

The court looks like a deep pit; brick walls rise up on all four sides. It is crowded below with school sinks, and these we found unspeakably filthy, with three weazened little chaps playing hide and seek between them. The ground floor of the house is a pork shop, where huge cauldrons of pork fat boil day and night. Even from the roof above we noticed the sickening odor. Inspecting the cellar, we found a strange odor of gas. The floor as usual was damp uneven earth. A huge sewer main ran along one side. In this we found three gaps the size of your fist, and . . . hence the odor, which mingled with the other odors in the pit outside.

Every form of human desperation throve in this atmosphere; nutrition was poor, alcoholism endemic, and consumption, particularly in a few buildings, rampant. As of the time Poole wrote, treatment of any sort was rare, and though registration of all cases was required in theory and laws were on the books requiring the forced segregation of recalcitrant consumptives, the sheer dimension of the problem made enforcement inconsistent at best. The stricken continued to work as long as they could—one Rumanian Jew Poole visited had, like most of his neighbors, begun labor at six in the morning and ended it at ten at night, persisting until he was no longer able to rise.

Denizens of the Lung Block tended to shy away from medical treatment even where it was available. Rumors circulated persistently of a black bottle, from which charity doctors were supposed to administer the coup de grace to hopeless cases. And later, as the city finally established facilities for consumptives, the intended beneficiaries balked, in many cases understandably. In 1902 the city opened a hospital for the "consumptive poor" and "moribund cases" on Blackwell's Island, run by the Department of Charities and Correction, the very pairing of titles suggesting, perhaps, why the poor viewed it with suspicion. It was joined in 1903 by a new facility, the Riverside Sanatorium for Pulmonary Diseases on North Brother Island.

Though called a sanatorium, the latter institution was designed, in the words of one of its proponents, for "wilfully careless consumptives under forcible detention." Its intended beneficiaries referred to it unceremoniously as the "consumptives' prison," and they regarded it with dread. Edwin S. Brown's 1922 novel, *The House of Strength* (mainly an account of the Modern Woodmen Sanatorium near Colorado Springs), describes in detail the terror the hospital inspired among the poor when Giovanni, his hero, learns he has tuberculosis and remembers seeing a lunger seized by the city police and dragged off, pleading but doomed, to Blackwell's Island. Poole, meeting a consumptive Lung Block mother and child, offered to set up a subscription to send them to the country for a cure, rather than to the city's hospital camps on the East River Islands, but the woman's response was characteristically hopeless. She expected death and saw no point in prolonging the agony in strange surroundings: "It's got to come anyway, an' we'd get homesick for the block, so I guess we'll stay."

To middle-class philanthropists appalled by slum life, it was incomprehensible that the poor might actually regard their neighborhoods with affection, and this very often became for the bemused benefactor a sign of ethnic inferiority and an excuse for administering charity with an iron hand. Inevitably, then, the drift of the socially conscious antituberculosis crusader, beginning in the 1890s and persisting at least through the prosperity of the 1920s (when in any case the mortality from consumption had begun to fall steeply), was in favor of compulsion. This began in school: hygiene teachers began to appear in the classroom, and children added health doxologies to their assignments for rote memory:

> I must keep my skin clean,
> Wear clean clothes,
> Breathe pure air,
> And live in the sunlight.

The leading American proponent of social control as a spearhead in the War on Tuberculosis was Hermann M. Biggs, and though his sphere of operation was confined to New York, he

became a figure of national importance in the movement, perhaps less publicized than Trudeau and Koch but more influential precisely because his main interest was the use of political
power. Science, Koch's tool, and practical doctoring, Trudeau's, were potent influences, and both lent themselves to
publicity. Legislation was a less seductive public topic, but its
influence was no less far-reaching. It was Biggs who, more than
any other single figure, led the movement to make illness not
just a fiefdom of science but a matter of law.

Compared to Koch and Trudeau his life was uneventful. He
was born in Trumansburg, New York, in 1859 to an unremarkable family in the hardware business and had an upbringing
notable, given later developments, for its devotion to planning. Biggs and his father used to execute contracts with each
other—one specified that the younger Biggs was to receive five
cents for every day he played the piano for an hour and that
he was to pay his father five cents for every day he didn't.
Another contract established a parentally administered savings account, to which little Hermann was to contribute one
dollar a month, earning interest at 10 percent per annum, but
forfeiting ten cents for every month he failed to make a deposit.

The passion for order this suggests followed Biggs through
his undergraduate years at Cornell, where he first conceived
an interest in public health and a conviction that it could be
bettered by sanitary reform. His baccalaureate thesis, on the
subject of sanitary science, was prescient in its appreciation of
the significance of Koch's discovery (a matter on which it was
in advance even of the American Medical Association, at
whose June 1882 national convention Koch was not even mentioned). But Biggs went beyond the science to a political consequence: if a disease had an indisputable factual basis, the social
consequences following from it were equally indisputable.
"Upon the recognition and careful observance of hygienic
laws," he wrote, "depend the healthy physical condition and
so the prosperity not only of individuals and communities, but
also of whole states and nations."

In 1883 Biggs took his M.D. from the Bellevue Medical College, from which he graduated at the head of his class; this too was fateful. The college was a bastion of clinical pathology—among its leading faculty were Francis Delafield and Edward Janeway (the renowned diagnostician who ten years before had treated Trudeau)—but it adapted readily to newer currents, and by the 1880s had begun to ride the new wave of bacteriological study. Perhaps still more important from Biggs's point of view, Bellevue had begun its institutional life in 1816 as a prison and was wedded from its earliest days as a hospital to the concept of supplying aid, sometimes forcibly, to the indigent.

Biggs's experience first as a student and young practitioner and later as a public health official further bred in him the conviction that the brightest future for medical endeavor lay not, as Koch would have supposed, in scientific discovery but in law. In 1888 he was appointed consulting pathologist to the city department of health, and in 1889 consulting physician to the Hospital for Contagious Diseases on North Brother Island.

On May 28, 1889, Biggs and his colleague T. M. Prudden submitted to the city of New York what was to prove an epoch-making report on the subject of tuberculosis. Like virtually every public and private statement Biggs was to make, it was direct and simple; he knew the value, when dealing with the public and their political representatives, of not clouding an issue with complications. The report made three forcible points about consumption, following from Koch: (1) it was preventable; (2) it was not inherited and not an expression of the constitution of the sufferer; and (3) it was caused by the tubercle bacillus, which was usually transmitted via dried and pulverized sputum carried through the air.*

From this Biggs and Prudden proposed for the city a three-pronged course of action: eliminate infected meat and milk

*All these points save the last were grounded in fact; it remains uncertain how important a medium dried sputum is, and current opinion seems to favor the theory that tuberculosis is most frequently carried by still-wet droplets of airborne saliva.

through a program of regular cattle inspection; disseminate widely to the population, through a publicity campaign, the knowledge that consumption was communicable and that the sputum of infected persons was hence dangerous; and systematically disinfect rooms and personal effects used by the tubercular.

Since, at the time, the city was enjoying the rule of a relatively enlightened and public-spirited administration, these reforms were quickly implemented. Leaflets in several languages were printed and distributed, giving nine points of advice about avoiding the contagion. Many of them were indisputable, but in view of later developments the sixth was particularly significant: "Do not fail to consult the family physician regarding the social relations of persons suffering from suspected consumption." For the program Biggs was beginning to imagine was nothing less than social engineering disguised as medicine. Over the next few years his attention was temporarily diverted from the conquest of tuberculosis: he turned his efforts to the founding of the world's first city-run pathological and bacteriological laboratory, and between 1894 and 1896 the laboratory devoted itself to an attack on diphtheria. Biggs spearheaded the American movement to use the newly discovered German diphtheria antitoxin, shepherding it through the inevitable controversies that surrounded its introduction in New York, and set up a scheme by which the New York City health department manufactured and distributed it to other cities who were without the resources to do so.

But Biggs soon returned to antituberculosis work, recommending in 1893 what was to become by far his most controversial antituberculosis measure. In addition to a repeated call for the dissemination of information to the public, Biggs now urged that all public institutions be required to transmit to the health department the names and addresses of anyone they encountered with tuberculosis. He also recommended setting up a corps of health inspectors to be dispatched to any building in which a case of consumption had occurred: "It shall be the duty of these inspectors to visit such premises and deliver proper circulars, and give suitable information, to the persons residing there, and take such specific measures of disinfection as are required in each case." Hospitals were henceforward encouraged to isolate tubercular patients; the Department of Charities and Correction was urged to establish a "Consumptive Hospital"; and all *private* physicians were "requested" to notify the health department of all cases of tuberculosis.

Some influential segments of public opinion approved heartily of these steps and saw in Biggs's mounting campaign no authoritarianism or hygienic hysteria. The press had, in the dozen years since Koch, gone from indifference or hostility to bacteriological research to histrionic advocacy. The *New York Sun* was particularly enthusiastic, remarking in an editorial on February 15, 1894: "The Board of Health formally declared war upon consumption when it adopted Professor Hermann Biggs's plan of campaign yesterday." And the prospect of introducing more formidable weapons to the arsenal did not trouble the paper. "The Board will not yet compel physicians to report their consumptive patients. That will come later on. It is the only thing that remains to be done, to put the worst of all contagious diseases into the column where it properly belongs."

At this point in his career Biggs's strategy was twofold: to enlist the press in arousing public concern, not to say panic, over the disease, and then to build upon that concern in a drive for more and more restrictive laws governing consumption and the consumptive. He was, in his popular writings, explicitly at pains to transfer some of the terror the public felt for acute illnesses to tuberculosis. In a piece entitled "To Rob Consumption of Its Terrors," he rather paradoxically argued, "If as many deaths occurred daily for one month from Asiatic cholera in New York as regularly occur from pulmonary consumption, the city would be well-nigh depopulated from the panic resulting." He then went on to suggest still more draconian public health measures: "the systematic employment of bacteriological examinations of the sputum for the early diagnosis of tuberculosis, [and] the enactment of regulations which shall forbid the employment of tubercular persons in such occupations as shall expose others to danger."

Bacteriology was, in Biggs's hands, being turned to purposes which its pioneers had never imagined. Very early in the history of medicine, of course, it had been realized that certain diseases were contagious and that their spread could be prevented by isolating those who had come down with the disease in question. But microbiology had, for the first time, supplied counters, traces, something definite to which the illness could be attributed. This in turn led to a new role for record keeping and testing; the progress of an epidemic could be tracked (if the rules were strict enough) as it spread from victim to victim, and the resulting increase in social control could be justified on the basis of simple fact. The microscope, in Biggs's hands, was becoming an instrument of power as well as inquiry, and the presence of a bacterium equivalent in its consequences to committing a felony.

By 1897 Biggs was advocating, and at least to some degree getting, more and more authority over the tubercular, their physicians, and even their dwelling places. The Blackwell's Island hospital opened, terrorizing the poor and powerless; but, perhaps unsurprisingly, it aroused less controversy than another, more far-reaching Biggs proposal: the compulsory registration of all cases of consumption. This set off a storm of protest; the loudest and most influential voice was the *Medical Record,* which editorialized succinctly:

> The real obnoxiousness of this amendment to the sanitary code is its offensively dictatorial and defiantly compulsory character. It places the Board in the rather equivocal position of dictating to the profession and creating a suspicion of an extra bid for public applause by unduly magnifying the importance of its bacteriological department.

Of course the outrage here is at the doctor's loss of authority, not at the patient's loss of privacy, but in another editorial the *Record* extended its concern to the victims of consumption: "It is . . . the extra missionary work assumed by the board which is the ominous and threatening quantity in the equation—the desire to assume official control of the cases after they have been reported."

Opposition did not intimidate Biggs; he continued to argue, more and more hotly, for even greater control. In 1900 he read a paper before the Philadelphia County Medical Society, again calling for registration. In it he dismissed, essentially without argument, all the objections to it, asserting among other dubious contentions that tuberculosis *was* casually transmissible and that the victim's fear of ostracism should his condition be publicized was "greatly exaggerated."

His most sweeping manifesto, however, had been issued three years before, in an address to the British Medical Association, meeting in Montreal, where he in effect argued that liberty ended at every threat, no matter how slight or how uncertain, to the public's health. Biggs defined health broadly.

> The government of the United States is democratic, but the sanitary measures adopted are sometimes autocratic, and the functions performed by sanitary authorities paternal in character. We are prepared, when necessary, to introduce and enforce, and the people are ready to accept, measures which might seem radical and arbitrary, if they were not plainly designed for the public good, and evidently beneficent in their effects. Even among the most ignorant of our foreign-born population, few or no indications of resentment are exhibited to the exercise of arbitrary powers in sanitary matters. The public press will approve, the people are prepared to support, and the courts sustain, any intelligent procedures which are evidently directed to the preservation of the public health.

The board of health in New York, according to Biggs, properly had powers as extensive as they were vaguely defined.

> The most autocratic powers, capable of the broadest construction, are given to them under the law. Everything which is detrimental to health or dangerous to life, under the freest interpretation, is regarded as coming within the province of the Health Department. So broad is the con-

struction of the law that everything which improperly or unnecessarily interferes with the comfort or enjoyment of life, as well as those things which are, strictly speaking, detrimental to health or dangerous to life, may become the subject of action on the part of the Board of Health.

Biggs was here communicating his vision of things as he wanted them to be rather than as they were. Perhaps fortunately for the personal freedom of New Yorkers, the Tammany Hall administration of Robert Van Wyck had come to power in 1897, and its preoccupation with the profitable business of clubhouse politics worked against any strong interest in benevolent large-scale social schemes. But when the Republicans returned to power in 1901, Biggs became general medical officer of the health department and once again found himself in a position to act on some cherished plans. In 1903 Biggs added a facility, the Riverside Sanatorium for Pulmonary Diseases on North Brother Island, to the one already established on Blackwell's Island.

Plans also went forward for the city's rural sanatorium at Otisville, which finally opened in 1905. Though not intended for the recalcitrant—the literature it passed out to prospective patients implied they had won a rare privilege in gaining admission to it—it still performed its charitable office with a Biggsean ardor. Biggs rebelled against the rationale of the rest cure, substituting a "work cure." This, he reasoned, would reduce costs, since inmates would be to some degree earning their keep; it would also serve "as a means of avoiding the cultivation of habits of idleness and in order to prepare the patients for subsequent self-support." As Biggs's assistant, Dr. Charles Boldman, explained it:

> There were individuals . . . whose lives were so worthless to the community that it would be an unpardonable waste of public funds to give them the benefit of sanatorium care. . . . [Biggs] objected to the "rest cure" enforced at various other sanatoria on the ground that their successful cases often consisted in "converting a sick tuberculous individual into a fairly healthy loafer."

At Otisville you embarked after the initial period of bed rest not merely on occupational therapy and exercise but on a useful trade, if possible the one you had followed before becoming ill. Though under its subsequent management Otisville somewhat abated the rigors of Biggs's plan for it, it kept his impress of muscular charity.

In fact Biggs never attained the sweeping arbitrary powers somewhat prematurely celebrated in his 1897 address to the British Medical Association. True, compulsory registration of tuberculosis cases came into being in New York (though widespread elsewhere, it never became universal); the hospital-prison at Riverside was built; and Otisville continued to practice its stern version of the cure. But Biggs had wanted all homebound consumptives placed under the direct supervision of the department of health and suggested as well that the system might be extended to those suffering from mental disorders. He proposed such measures at the ninth annual meeting of the National Association for the Study and Prevention of Tuberculosis in 1913, where, happily, they languished.

In fact, the antituberculosis movement successfully resisted the impulse toward compulsory treatment; the spirit of Trudeau prevailed, and in the end the nation by and large treated consumption the way Saranac Lake treated it. A few laws were enacted, but the core of the effort was voluntary. The public's fear of consumption was to be allayed through a massive publicity campaign representing the disease as curable and promising, in the most optimistic of the slogans, the eradication of tuberculosis by 1914. The victim's fear of hospitalization was to be assuaged by making the sanatorium as pleasant a place as possible; good sanitary habits were fostered by education rather than by ordinance. Members of the medical profession, perhaps under the moderating influence of the lay volunteers in the movement, resisted the impulse to convert their authority into hegemony; and in the end persuasion and trust proved stronger than statutory power. In his book *Authority,* Richard Sennett has pointed out that power comes not from the authority's ability to compel but from the trust we place in those who wield it. It forges an inner bond stronger than the coercive one Biggs would have established, as it doesn't depend on enforcement, and thus doesn't invite rebellion.

Biggs went on to become commissioner of the New York State Health Department in 1913. Its powers were growing as New York began to establish a statewide system of sanatoriums, all of which had to be supervised. The post was an ideal one for Biggs, in that it suited his drive for control, and probably also for the tuberculosis movement, since it placed him at one remove from the treatment of patients—he was using statutes to boss county health boards and state bureaucrats rather than inflicting himself directly on the ill, as he had been doing in New York City. Yet under his aegis the state established an exemplary antituberculosis plan, and by the 1930s virtually every county operated its own sanatorium; there were, besides, three state hospitals. They were well organized; but most of them were far gentler in spirit than was the early Otisville.

Laws, in other words, never became the principal vehicles of the social wing of the last crusade; de Tocqueville's observation that Americans much preferred voluntary efforts marshaled by interested parties had proved apt. Of course, some laws, encouraged by the antituberculosis movement—those designed to encourage better housing, better food supplies, better medical care generally—were in many cases put on the books under its pressure. But they were fragments of the picture, important but deceptive in that they distort the essential feature of the campaign. The ferocious Biggs was an exception to a general blurring of lines between professional medicine and lay activism, legislation and voluntarism, between doctor and patient, between the scientific and the popular. Early in American history de Tocqueville had noticed the republic's taste for associations, people from different walks of life gathered together in the service of a good cause:

Americans of all ages, all conditions, and all dispositions constantly form associations. They have not only commercial and manufacturing companies, in which all take part, but associations of a thousand other kinds, religious, moral, serious, futile, general or restricted, enormous or diminutive. The Americans make associations to give entertainments, to found seminaries, to build inns, to construct churches, to diffuse books, to send missionaries to the antipodes; in this manner they found hospitals, prisons, and schools. If it is proposed to inculcate some truth or to foster some feeling by the encouragement of a great example, they form a society.

Such associations, de Tocqueville observed, often initiated by men of rank, exercised a power over social policy just short of official status, yet far more sweeping than one might at first expect from an informal union of interested parties.

No facet of the War on Consumption reflects this phenomenon better than the Framingham and Syracuse demonstrations. Both were attempts to create in miniature a state-of-the-art health crusade, pooling the talents of doctors, social engineers, community planners, private enterprise, and average citizens. In both cities the aim was to marshal all available civic resources for a concerted attack on consumption rather than, as in earlier campaigns, trusting to the uncoordinated efforts of various voluntary groups like the local antituberculosis societies.* The plan went beyond a mere assault on the disease; the aim was rather to change the way citizens thought about it, indeed to change the way they lived. And though public health laws were part of the plan, coercion was in the main both more subtle and more widespread, relying as it did on persuasion, social pressure, and the careful fostering of apparently spontaneous public enthusiasm.

*At the commencement of its pioneering experiment in 1916, Framingham had about sixteen thousand citizens, population enough to function as an urban center but small enough to make control of the experiment easy. Syracuse, whose program began seven years later, was at the time a city twelve times as big, and its program was an attempt to apply the principles of the Framingham demonstration, just then ending, in a larger metropolis.

The Framingham experiment began not in government but private enterprise, in the Metropolitan Life Insurance Company in New York. In 1915 the company observed that 14,325 of its policyholders had died of tuberculosis; it had paid out $4 million in claims on their lives. Lee K. Frankel, a company physician, discussed this problem with a number of leading figures in the antituberculosis movement, and on May 3, 1916, Frankel wrote to E. R. Baldwin (then medical director at the Trudeau Sanatorium and president of the national association) with a proposal. The company would donate $100,000 for a three-year experiment in a town of five thousand people (the population limit was later raised, the study extended from three years to seven, and the contribution by the Metropolitan raised to roughly $183,000) in New York or Massachusetts, the states where the largest plurality of the company's policyholders lived and where antituberculosis activity was already fairly well developed.

As Frankel envisioned it, the first goal was to encourage periodic medical examinations for every member of the community; to supply proper medical care for the tubercular, in sanatoriums where necessary, and through a dispensary where that was impossible; and in the service of these goals to enlist "the cooperation of local and state health officers, employers, labor unions, school authorities, etc." The national association was to oversee the experiment, working as far as possible through the community's own leaders. "How," the question was, "can social forces best be used to prevent unnecessary sickness and death, particularly from tuberculosis?"

As soon as the national association had accepted Metropolitan Life's offer and Framingham was selected as the pilot program's site, committees began to sprout and proliferate. These included a national committee (consisting of influential figures in the antituberculosis movement and community leaders); an executive staff, hired to supervise the experiment; and a flotilla of local committees—a committee of local members of the national committee, a fourteen-member local executive committee, a 130-member advisory council charged with educating the public, "an Exclusion Committee designed to detect an invasion of the community by the migratory consumptive," an industrial health committee, an infant welfare committee; finally, at the grass roots, "neighborhood committees, selected on a block basis, representative of the leading personalities in the community, to serve as a direct channel of interchange between the Health Demonstration office and the homes of the people, as an instrument for the gradual taking of a social inventory of the community, etc."

Whatever separately charged with, together these committees were meant to gather information. Saranac Lake grew naturally, even stumbled, into its modus vivendi with tuberculosis; Framingham was to achieve the same result by study. The committees gathered statistics about tuberculosis in the town for the ten years before 1917. They studied rural and urban sanitary conditions, milk production and handling, school hygiene, and working conditions in local factories. Most intensely and most systematically, though, they studied the townspeople. Tuberculin tests were given to all children between one and seven years old (33.3 percent of these tested positive, 66.7 percent negative). Families with a history of tuberculosis were to be subjected to intense scrutiny, since "light must be thrown, if possible, on the relative importance of infection on the one hand, and hereditary resistance on the other." And, finally, a survey of economic and social conditions would be made as part of a "Patriotic Census": leading citizens from every district in the town would dig out vital facts about Framingham's home hygiene.* Local doctors were recruited,

---

*World War I broke out just as the antituberculosis crusade was coming of age. At first this caused some apprehension among the movement's leaders—should they, perhaps, defer to the war effort? Eventually they concluded that public health was even more important in wartime than during peace: the national stock of healthy young men had to be kept up. So instead of folding, the campaign expanded, adopting in the process a stock of war imagery that it was never to discard. And the mobilization of national opinion in favor of the war effort, and in favor of the antituberculosis movement, came to reinforce each other. Both were, after all, case studies in the molding of mass opinion.

alerted to the threat of consumption, and encouraged to examine their patients more carefully for signs of latent or cryptic infection. Nurses and "insurance agents from the several larger companies" were to fan out through the town in a "health/sickness canvass," performed at the beginning and the end of the experiment. Insurance agents were to screen those families insured by their companies; nurses were to interview the uninsured.

A leaflet was distributed throughout the town, explaining the census, and asking cooperation: *"Health First for Framingham—All Else Will Follow."* Each investigator got a supply of preprinted cards on which to enter information (the Framingham Demonstration became a prodigious spawner of forms) and a booklet of instructions.

But all this was a mere preface to the centerpiece of the campaign, the mass medical examination. The aim was to transform the town's image of the checkup; no longer an extraordinary procedure, it was to be thought of as an annual routine. Good for the townspeople, who would, once steeped in the habit, detect illnesses early while they were still amenable to treatment. Good also for the insurance company, spared the paying out of avoidable claims; good, of course, for the physician. During the health census, all surveyed families were asked if they would submit to a free physical examination. On April 17, 1917, a notice appeared in the *Framingham Evening News,* announcing that the newly formed Community Health Station would offer, to *"the first 500 Framingham families applying,* a free, thorough medical examination by experts, who will examine families in their homes, and recommend sick persons discovered to their own *Framingham doctors for treatment."* Like much of the early propaganda in the campaign, this advertisement invoked the war effort: "COMMUNITY HEALTH IS ESSENTIAL TO NATIONAL PREPAREDNESS. NOW IS THE TIME TO SHOW THAT WASTEFUL SICKNESS CAN BE PREVENTED." Churches were persuaded to pass out notices on the Sunday before the first drive. The town blossomed with leaflets passed out by insurance men, doctors, nurses, and Boy

Scouts. All was voluntary, however, the Biggs spirit avoided:
physicians were instructed, for example, to avoid shows of
authority: "You may find that while a family has previously
agreed to the medical examination, they have since changed
their minds. In that instance, simply make a record of this on
the Examination Record and withdraw pleasantly."

But the publicity was so widespread, the canvassing and
recanvassing so persistent, that they bordered on intimidation.
Families who missed their home examinations were summoned by special messenger to the Health Station on Union
Avenue. Each person examined received a "popularly worded
medical examination diagnosis and treatment record." Anyone found sick was urged to seek treatment from a local doctor; anyone positively diagnosed, or suspected of being tubercular, endured "nursing visits, re-examinations, sputum
examinations, temperature observation, X-ray, and other measures, until a definite classification of the case could be made."

The examination campaign lasted twenty-four days, em-
ployed forty-odd physicians (some donated their time, but
most were paid $5.00 or $10.00 per session), and took in 4,473
people, over a quarter of the population, at a final cost of $1.84
per person. The results of these examinations were startling:
77 percent of the examinees were reported to be ill.

The method by which these figures emerged tells a good
deal about the mentality of the public health fraternity at the
time. Diseases were divided into three categories: "Preventable or Easily Remediable," "Doubtfully Preventable," and
"Nonpreventable." There appears to have been a strong pre-
disposition first in favor of finding a large number of illnesses,
then of finding most of these preventable. The 6,167 different
incidences of sickness the examiners found included 1,520
cases of bad teeth, 1,148 of enlarged tonsils, and 96 of tuberculosis, all lumped together as "preventable." There were also
243 colds ("doubtfully preventable"). Only 877 of the reported
ailments were adjudged nonpreventable, and these were divided into subgroups so vague as to be nearly meaningless as
diagnoses: cardiac, cardiovascular, renal, vascular, and

"other." If one subtracted colds, bad teeth, and sore throats from the total, the illness quotient shrank spectacularly. Though the focus of the demonstration was a major life-threatening disease, the public health movement regarded all indispositions as evils to be combated. Toothaches and colds were not routine ailments to be lived with cheerfully; they were linked with the enemy under assault.

The ninety-six cases of tuberculosis uncovered represented about 2 percent of the people examined. There were twenty-five cases of incipient, seventeen of advanced, and fifty-four of arrested disease; ten of these people eventually left town for treatment at a sanatorium or comparable institution. The Italian population proved generally resistant to consumption; the Irish and French Canadians disproportionately susceptible. Income and living conditions turned out not to be as decisive a factor in the disease as the investigators had anticipated.

From this welter of surveys, examinations, and statistics, the leaders of the program moved on to measures they thought of as practical. The tubercular were tracked as carefully as troops in the war. Every Framingham consumptive was identified by a pin bearing the date of his diagnosis. As his condition bettered or worsened the pin moved backward or forward on a large chart divided into columns: "Suspicious," "Early," "Advanced," "Arrested," "Moved," or "Dead." The contagious were urged to seek treatment at sanatoriums; other victims were, where possible, treated at home, sometimes after a brief hospital stay, intended as much for its educational as its clinical effects. Children exposed to tuberculosis at home were, where possible, sent to live with foster families. "Incorrigible" cases were monitored, urged, pleaded with, hectored, threatened, and eventually treated by whatever arrangements they would submit themselves to. But they were not forced into hospitals; there was no tuberculosis prison.

Except insofar as the whole town was incarcerated in a grid of volunteers. Committees descended on schools and factories in search of unsanitary conditions, poor ventilation, and other threats to health. The schools were found wanting in all categories: rooms were overheated, indifferently lit, and poorly furnished. Between one third and two thirds of the factories showed poor hygienic conditions—dirty floors, poor lighting and ventilation, fumes, hazardous substances, and poor sanitary facilities.

Framingham founded a summer day camp on an abandoned fairground on the outskirts of the town. It was not meant for children actually suffering from consumption but rather for those "exposed to tuberculous infection and those who are under-par, anemic, physically defective, badly nourished, under weight and undersize." The campers were fed amply—two lunches were served at 10:30 A.M. and 3:45 P.M., including hearty items like egg sandwiches, peanut butter, tapioca, and chocolate cornstarch pudding. During the week of August 4, 1919, the children dutifully consumed 405,125 calories, at a cost of seventeen cents per child. Between meals they played, rested, swam, waded, underwent Toothbrush Drill, and listened to lectures on hygiene and good diet.

In 1917 the 116 homes from which the attending children had come were visited and carefully evaluated by project workers. Nearly half of them, according to the resulting survey, were either "fair" or "bad" as to cleanliness. Eighty-two percent of the houses had flies, 40 percent had mosquitoes. In 73 percent there was no provision for outdoor sleeping (compare Saranac Lake, where by this date virtually all houses had one or more sleeping porches), and in 76 percent of the homes the children did not sleep alone. Seventy percent of them had what the volunteers determined were fair or bad hygienic habits. The nurse who visited each child's home was given a form to guide her inquiry; it covered the house itself, the family's health habits, the personal hygiene of the child. "Habits . . . Bathes weekly . . . Care of mouth . . . Hands . . . Food: amount . . . kinds . . . tea . . . coffee . . . milk . . . regular . . . well cooked . . . satisfactory breakfast . . . supper . . . How spends time . . . hours in bed . . . sleeps alone . . . sleeps out . . . Work: hours . . . place . . . kind . . . condition . . . mentally sound . . . cooperative . . ."

An account of the Framingham Demonstration may well be numbing to read, but its effect on the participants must have been different. From beginning to end it was an exercise not in actual coercion but in incessant benevolent surveillance and gentle nagging. Very little was done; nobody was ever forced into anything. But the citizens were prodigiously asked things, reminded of things; the project amassed not political power but information. Without punitive laws or crude interference, the town was being gently badgered into an awareness of tuberculosis. Every Saturday for three years the *Evening News* gave over a column to a weekly health letter. "How Can We Fight Tuberculous Infection?" "How Can We Fight Tuberculous Disease?" "How Can We Reduce Deaths from Tuberculosis?" The same few facts reappeared again and again in new guises, like "The Tuberculosis Catechism."

The keystone of all this publicity was neither sanatorium treatment nor hygiene (though both were important); it was the regular medical examination. Surely this was the first time the need for preventive medical inspection was drummed so persistently into the public mind, in an effort to make people do willingly what Biggs wanted to force them into, as the following advertisement shows:

Your Annual Medical Examination!!
Have You Had It?
It May Add Years to Your Life!
Why is machinery inspected regularly?
Why do we overhaul our automobiles?
BECAUSE IT PAYS!
The "human machine" is a most delicate device, and it needs an inspection and adjustment occasionally, if it is not to be scrapped before its time.
A THOROUGH EXAMINATION
1. Will find correctible defects—and save future misery.
2. Will increase your physical efficiency and happiness.
3. Will detect fatal disease, curable only in the *beginning stages,* such as cancer.
4. *Will find tuberculosis in time!*

But in 1923 the demonstration and its attendant harangues came to an end. Medical examinations had indeed become a routine feature of the average citizen's year; health education had been made the center of the town's public life; Framingham knew which of its inhabitants were well, which sick, and why. Over the seven years of the project, the death rate from tuberculosis had fallen 68 percent, a far steeper drop than was occurring in the state at large (the control town for the experiment showed a drop of 32 percent). And all this had been achieved without coercion and without a crushing capital investment. The guiding lights behind the experiment had divined that the forces of public health would be stronger if they worked by persuasion; voluntary compliance was a stronger force than law, and the people behind the project were persuaded that psychology was their most powerful health weapon. The anonymous writer of the final 1923 report on the project put it succinctly:

> In this work the psychological appeals through which an individual might be urged to submit to a health examination were most varied. A small but important nucleus of the community was interested in the work from the scientific angle. . . . A somewhat larger group was interested in *Framingham* and was moved to participation by a local patriotic animus. Another group was made up of those, particularly among the foreign born, who were willing to take something for nothing, the health examination being free. Perhaps the most important group of all numerically was those who had a definite and logical and personal selfish interest in the matter, who thought they might have something the matter with them and wanted to find out what it was. Finally, a fairly important middle-class group, following the trail of the scientific or community minded individuals enumerated first above, on a largely imitative basis, participated in the health examination campaign, this being "the thing to do."

Framingham's example was imitated. In 1923 the Milbank Memorial Fund decided to sponsor a project modeled on the Framingham experiment, this time in a larger city, Syracuse, New York.

By 1923 Syracuse had grown from a swampy flat near Onondaga Lake, dismal enough "to make an owl weep to fly over it" to an industrial city of two hundred thousand. It had a good water supply, adequate sanitation, and decent but not exceptional facilities for health care. The Milbank grant aimed at a larger-scale repetition of the Framingham modus operandi: consciousnesses were to be raised, voluntary efforts coordinated, the city steeped in knowledge about tuberculosis, and steeled to combat it. Studies were conducted, and the city was encouraged to increase its health appropriations. Two new tuberculosis nurses were hired; seminars on the disease were organized for physicians. Schoolchildren were examined; a publicity campaign materialized. Coercion was avoided; voluntary participation was, as at Framingham, the watchword. As at Framingham, the tuberculosis death rate plummeted significantly, though this plunge was not much more dramatic than the fall in death rates throughout New York State during the same period.

As at the sanatorium, so in the cities and towns: the antituberculosis movement depended more on insinuating itself as a way of life than on the grosser interferences of law and statute. It was a crusade that spent its effort, from the opening of the first sanatoriums through the dawn of the antibiotic era during World War II, as much on influencing the way people thought as on attacking the tubercle bacillus.

That such campaigns did not fall on deaf ears is nowhere clearer than in the enthusiasm with which the forces of business embraced them. It became a matter of good public relations as well as an expression of corporate benevolence for businesses to monitor the lungs of their employees. Companies such as Metropolitan Life Insurance, which gave its workers yearly examinations and dispatched the ailing for a free stay at its Mount McGregor Sanatorium, and Standard Oil, with its pavilion at the Loomis Sanatorium, built exclusively for the use of its tubercular employees, were not the exception. Stony Wold Sanatorium, founded near Saranac Lake in 1903 for indigent women and children, became a retreat for consumptive telephone operators, largely supported by the New York Telephone Company.

These, of course, were all reputable enterprises, conducted strictly in conformity with orthodox medical practice and approved by the medical and social magisterium of the national association. But in one sense the potency of the movement the latter group began is attested to by the rapidity with which it escaped orthodox control and kindled the interest of ambitious mavericks. The War on Tuberculosis had struck too resonant a chord to be confined to the professionals; enthusiasts chimed in.

Of these there were dozens, perhaps hundreds. Patent medicines, for instance, chased from the marketplace by the forces of reason, returned incorrigibly in answer to the needs of panic. In 1904 the United States Senate held a hearing on fraudulent "rejuvenators" and tuberculosis cures; the Post Office pressed fraud cases, frequently and often futilely, against mail-order cures, whose most frequent targets were cancer, consumption, and epilepsy. "Tubercleicide" appeared in 1916. Because its main ingredient, creosote carbonate, was thought by some reputable physicians to be effective against the disease, it hung on until 1928, when the Postmaster General finally succeeded in suppressing it. But "B & M External Remedy," sold by Frank E. Rollins, showed a vampire's longevity. The compound (comprised mainly of turpentine, ammonia, and raw eggs) had begun life as a horse liniment, but Rollins applied it to his tuberculous daughter, sister-in-law, and grandmother with, he claimed, miraculous results.

> White Plague Conquered!!! . . . The New Chemical Compound B & M External Remedy Has Won the Victory—Tubercular Germs are entirely eradicated from the lungs, glands, or joints in four to twelve weeks . . . without any change in mode of life. The breadwinner need not abandon his employment. . . . The expensive sanatorium treatment during months or years is no longer necessary.

The B & M regimen had its adherents. Mrs. Edith Merchant of Ashland, New Hampshire, for example, swore by it and offered to write a personal testimonial to any skeptic who applied (Rollins gratefully supplied her with a desk, stationery, stamps, and $1143.10); she kept this up indefatigably until, as her son regretfully informed Rollins, she died of tuberculosis. But B & M External Remedy survived until 1932.

Patent remedies for consumption had been common, of course, throughout the nineteenth century, but the generation that arose in the twenties and thirties struck a new note: they co-opted the imagery of the orthodox antituberculosis crusade, recognizing a powerful force when they saw it. The B & M promotional literature speaks of the cure as a "victory"; that term would never have occurred to Piso or Helmbold in the 1870s, when the treatment of consumption had not acquired the vocabulary of warfare. Tubercle bacilli, unknown in 1880, still dim in the popular imagination twenty years later, were, by 1920, minute villains, effective characters in popular advertising. The sanatorium cure had taken the place of Brand X as the rival remedy to be discredited. And yet, of course, even mentioning it familiarly placed B & M External Remedy subtly in its company, as if on a par with it.

There were hundreds of what James Harvey Young calls medical messiahs. But none was more influential, more irrepressible, or more plainly influenced by the antituberculosis movement than Bernarr MacFadden. Better, perhaps, than any other folk health hero, he illustrates just how deep the ethic of the Outdoor Life had sunk in the American psyche. His passion was health, or "Physical Culture," as he called it; but, not surprisingly, his business was mass-circulation publishing—*Physical Culture* itself, his brainchild and lifelong obsession, *True Story, Liberty,* and the New York *Graphic* (dubbed, by its detractors, the *Pornographic*).

He was born near Mill Springs, Missouri, in 1868, to, he said, an alcoholic father and a consumptive mother; when she died, little Bernarr was sent to work at a hotel near Chicago run by relatives, where, according to his official biographer, he reportedly overheard an exchange that was to affect the course of his life:

"Died o' consumption, Elizabeth did. I could see it. She had it a long time."

"Yep, I noticed how sickly she looked, when she wuz here."

"That brat o' hers is got it too. I never seen such a weakly, spindlin'-lookin'—"

"He'll go the same way she did, no doubt o' that."

He left the hotel to work on a farm; in his memory the life outdoors there and the heavy physical exertion proved his savior; a subsequent stint in Saint Louis at indoor work brought more deterioration; but joining a gymnasium and hiking the local countryside with weights strapped to his body reversed the slide. MacFadden became, then, in the 1880s, a firm devotee of strenuous exercise and a wholesome diet as infallible routes to good health and as specifics against consumption.

For the next few years he knocked about the Midwest, lifting weights and dabbling in various trades. He worked on a newspaper in McCune, Kansas, ran a gymnasium and a laundry, worked as a circus acrobat and a professional wrestler (all businesses that, save perhaps the laundry, were to stand him in good stead later on); but he knew his true calling long before he was able to make a living out of it:

Bernarr MacFadden
Kinisitherapist
Teacher of
Higher Physical Culture

He taught himself to write and speak in public and moved to New York, where, finding no publisher willing to market his manifestos and no manufacturer willing to sell the exercise machinery he had designed to accompany them, he decided to publish and sell both his prose and his machinery on his own. The project began with a fateful publicity tour to England. It was on this trip that he met his future wife, Mary Wellington.

An athletic young woman from Halifax, Yorkshire, she had won MacFadden's "Perfect Woman" contest, and he was so taken with her talents that he prevailed upon her to join his traveling Physical Culture demonstration, which played various provincial theaters to sometimes tumultuous audience response. The show was designed to demonstrate the virtues and attractions of Physical Culture, with MacFadden himself in various muscular poses as its proudest achievement. Initially, Mary's role was limited. As the orchestra played Chopin's Funeral March, MacFadden, clad only in a loincloth, lay down on his back on the stage floor; Mary portentously climbed from a chair to a table, from which, after a dramatic pause, she jumped onto MacFadden's stomach, bounced off its resilient muscles, then executed a few triumphant dance steps as MacFadden leapt to his feet and bowed in the spotlight. Together they were billed as "The World's Healthiest Man and Woman," and before long romance dawned.

They were married in 1913 and returned to the United States after a successful British tour. MacFadden began preaching the gospel of Physical Culture to his native country, which had, during earlier attempts, turned a deaf ear on him. That gospel was a populist parody of the Outdoor Life, an echo of the imagery of health successfully put across by the antituberculosis crusade. MacFadden sold, for example, a watch, festooned at the appropriate hours with instructions for healthful activities:

> Seven A.M. Wake up! Stretch! Rise quickly. Fifteen minutes' exercise. Deep breathing at open window. Douse in cold tub. Sing! Rough towel rub. Stay nude as long as possible.
>
> Eight A.M. No breakfast. Take glass cool water. . . . Walk to work. Identify the birds. Start day cheerfully!
>
> Ten A.M. Glass of milk or water. Never use ice. Noon. First meal. Eat slowly. Count 150 chews per mouthful. Chew tough foods. Don't drink at meals. Exercise teeth on tough sour bread. Prevents tooth decay.
>
> Noon to 5 P.M. Refuse to be rushed. Maintain cheerful mind.
>
> Five to six P.M. End of work. Five-mile walk with deep breathing. Rest before dinner. Count chews.

Eight to nine fifty-five. Don't work evenings. Have harmless time. Few nuts or grapes.

Ten P.M. Open windows wide. Let body breathe nude. Exercise until tired. Go to bed.

The insistence on regular habits, abundant fresh air, appropriate exercise, even more the emphasis on the importance of good cheer, was familiar from the antituberculosis crusade, and from the other components of the health movement as well. But MacFadden distilled the ideas, popularized them, and turned them into a creed. In the first editorial in *Physical Culture,* founded just after his return from Europe, MacFadden laid down the theory from which he was never to deviate. It reads like a parody of a sanatorium prospectus:

> Weakness is a crime. . . . One has no more excuse for being weak, than for going hungry, when food is at hand. . . . Disease is a result of the victim's own ignorance or carelessness. . . . Vigorous, pulsating [*sic*] health is within the reach of all.

MacFadden's creed took some rigorous forms. His remedy for toothache, for example, was to chew on a piece of wood, as a means of giving the teeth "a form of vigorous massage," preferring oak or mahogany over softer woods like pine. During his days at the laundry, his business partner had mistakenly thrown a dress with a bustle into the washing machinery, and the resulting wreckage gave MacFadden a lifelong distaste for excess in costume. Shoes, he believed, were bad for the feet; he often walked barefoot from his home in Nyack to his Manhattan office. He wore ventilated hats, remained nude whenever possible, and according to Mary MacFadden, execrated pajamas. "Pants in bed, he said, were a sinister invention calculated to thwart the inspirational moment of procreation."

Physical Culture never achieved the success MacFadden wanted for it, but it became the basis of a business whose other publications, especially *True Story,* made him a millionaire and allowed him to continue preaching his creed via every available medium to anyone who would, or would not, listen. He made a series of Physical Culture movies, including *Zontar*, *False Pride*, *Broken Homes*, and *Wives at Auction*. Imitating the health regimens of John Harvey Kellogg, he rented a vacant sanatorium in Battle Creek from C. W. Post and took in cancer patients, first experimenting with a milk cure, then moving on when it failed to an all-grape diet. In Chicago he founded the "Healthatorium," an institution for a time devoted to the theory that since humans had once walked on all fours, languishing health could be restored by a course of walking on one's knees and knuckles. He concocted and sold, with minimal success, a breakfast cereal, "Strenthro," also known as "Vigor Breakfast Grits." He opened a Health Home in upstate New York for invalids suffering from consumption, rheumatism, and paralysis and opened a Physical Culture City near Spottswood, New Jersey, where he offered to an obdurately uninterested nation a series of ideas meant to improve its health and its convenience.

It only stood to reason that, having cured himself of consumption through Physical Culture, MacFadden should try to persuade other consumptives to do likewise; in 1908 and 1909 he wrote a series of five articles on the disease in successive numbers of *Physical Culture* magazine. "It might," he says, "be termed a civilized malady for it is usually found among so-called civilized people," a disease of citified corruption, much less likely to strike in the pure air of the country. Mac-Fadden acknowledges the tubercle bacillus and bacteriology only to wave them confidently away:

> The victims of this terrible malady in many instances have an idea that they have acquired the complaint from another sufferer; that the tubercular bacilli have in some way been inhaled and from this minute beginning the disease has developed. This conclusion is in nearly all cases erroneous.

According to *Physical Culture*, the cause of consumption is rather low "vital resistance," which allows "catarrh of the nasal passages" to move down into the lungs: "it is impossible for a strong man to be attacked by consumption."

MacFadden's remedies for the disease, outlined in his remaining articles, were merely intensified versions of his prescriptions for general vitality and good health. Fresh air was most useful: "with every draught of air inhaled there is a wave of electrical energy which is distributed throughout the physical organism." "Coffee, and tea, meat, white bread, hot biscuits," on the other hand, are all "prominent causes of the lessened vitality which often results in consumption" and should be avoided. In the June and July 1909 issues, MacFadden advised consumptive readers to wear fewer clothes and embark on a program of vigorous stimulative exercise, including walks, running, and workouts with dumbbells. Exercise would be improved if accompanied by sun baths, air baths, cold water baths, and dry friction baths: "it is much better to take this dry friction bath with brushes as it is more valuable than using a rough towel." And finally the mind, the most powerful factor in restoring health, should be kept resolutely chipper. "Don't worry. Cultivate a hopeful attitude. Simply determine that health will be yours and begin to work for it with an indomitable determination."

MacFadden made his career as an indignant rebel against convention; however eccentric he may have been there was nothing of the hypocrite in him. He believed passionately in the superiority of Physical Culture over the therapies of orthodox medicine and squandered a good part of his publishing fortune on the effort to prove it. Yet, granted that central fact, it's curious how much his movement absorbed from current theories in established medicine and how much it obviously owed to the culture of the sanatorium movement. The technology MacFadden testily rejected; the imagery he wholeheartedly embraced. Fresh air, good food, a healthy cheerfulness of mind were his great enthusiasms; shedding the protections of city life and placing yourself open to the elemental forces of nature was his program; Physical Culture City and his various Healthatoria and sanatoria attest to his urge to enshrine these principles in ideal communities.

The thought that health might belong to a class of experts, adept in a lore inaccessible to everyone else, enraged him, and for the next twenty years he kept *Physical Culture* charging valiantly at the windmills of science. *"No disease* of whatever nature, name or kind, ever was or ever can be spread by contagion," Dr. M. J. Rodermund, an enthusiastic MacFadden acolyte, virtually shouted in a manifesto in the September 1909 issue. And even in the 1920s it was still doing battle with the germ theory of disease, though it occasionally allowed space to writers with other ideas. (Linda Burfield, D.O., wrote an article in the December 1920 issue, suggesting that tuberculosis was indeed probably caused by germs, but that these could be starved out if the invalid spent twenty-four days ingesting only water.) MacFadden was suspicious of expertise; he far preferred medical strategies anyone could master. "Remedying Self-Poisoning Constipation" was a typical article; so was "Dangers of a Big Stomach." (The latter included a photo with the following caption: "Side view of a fat man, showing the useless and needless load that he carries all through life.") Readers of *Physical Culture* were exhorted to shape up, think clean thoughts, eat simply, and were promised in turn that health would come to them as of right; populist as the approach was, it grew close enough to contemporary orthodox medicine to remain in its penumbra.

It was thus scarcely surprising that when the Loomis Sanatorium fell on hard times in the late 1930s and finally closed in 1938, a victim of declining patient populations, MacFadden should have been interested in it; he took the unused property over in 1944 and ran it until 1948 as a charitable institution, operating on MacFaddenesque principles. Eccentric though these were, they were not incompatible with, and not unconnected to, the orthodox sanatorium regimes. Clement Wood, his authorized biographer, summed up MacFadden's philosophy. Barring the theoretical underpinnings and occasional leaps into enthusiasm, Trudeau would have concurred in most of it:

He is against the city, and in favor of the country type of life. The very air of the city is devitalizing; the cities would die in a few generations without the transfusion of fresh country blood. He favors hard work for boys; is against leisure, unless it be capitalized into bodily and mental improvement; recommends suffering and hardship; . . . intelligent saving; . . . is against an excess of laws—the farmer is scornful of any regulations contrary to the ways things have always been done on the farm. He faces every problem that rises with that native shrewdness that grows among our farm population, and is a different thing from the quick-wittedness in overcoming the other fellow that marks the city product.

With MacFadden, the health movement returned with a vengeance to the common man and common sense, from which, in part, it had sprung. He reflected its enthusiasms, and, without the control of the public health movement exerted on them, those enthusiasms ran wild. But they attest to the pervasiveness of the public health movement in general and the crusade against tuberculosis on the other; both went beyond influencing the medical profession and the law. Nothing attests better to its influence than its power to inspire cranks.

8

"Some Vague, Awful Thing":
Novels, Plays, and Films

The bare fact was that Ratso did not look okay. Joe
was willing enough to lie about it and let the matter
pass, but something else happened as he continued to
look into Ratso's face.
What was it?
Neither of them really knew.
Some vague, awful thing had come into evidence
between them like a skeleton dancing on threads,
something grim and secret that filled Joe with terror,
making him feel locked out and alone and in peril.
—JAMES LEO HERLIHY,
Midnight Cowboy, 1965

Ratso Rizzo has tuberculosis; it is the shadow that haunts both
James Leo Herlihy's 1965 novel and the movie with Jon Voight
and Dustin Hoffman, made a few years later. Yet in neither the
picture nor the book does the shadow ever emerge into the
light. Both date from a decade after the closing of the sanatoriums, the triumph of antibiotics, and the emergence of the
nation from under the pall of the White Plague. Yet both
presume, despite the disappearance of consumption as a familiar disease, that the audience will recognize it, and moreover
not simply as a medical condition but one carrying universally
recognized—and by the standards of the antituberculosis crusade, rather archaic—metaphorical resonances.

Ratso is plainly decrepit on first appearance, though not
clearly tubercular. He's crippled, scrawny, furtive, hyperactive, entirely urban. These are, of course, all characteristics
connected subliminally with popular ideas of tuberculosis, but
the only unmistakable symptom in either book or movie is
Ratso's cough. It appears early, as Ratso leads the heedless Joe
to his first swindle, then rapidly worsens. He blames it on a

cold, then the flu. The book adds the information that he had had pneumonia and polio as a child; the movie, which makes Ratso's father a shoeshine man, has Ratso remember a nagging cough, which he attributes to the irritating effects of shoe polish.

Film and book are both assiduous in not mentioning tuberculosis. Ratso and Joe are equally determined, and their reluctance seems poised between simple ignorance and a knowledgeable fear of naming something dreaded; in fact they quarrel over a name for it. "Joe wanted to call it cat fever, a name Sally [his grandmother] had liked to apply to a number of disorders he'd suffered in childhood on the theory that all sicknesses came from cats, but Ratso said he hadn't been *near* a cat, and besides, what he had was the flu."

One by one the symptoms accumulate—the cough, the pallor, the night sweats, the advancing weakness. Perhaps even more important, so do all the mythological echoes a hundred years of cultural history had struck off consumption. Ratso, living in abandoned tenements; dreams of moving to a better climate, away from the city crowds. In the film, Joe instinctively brings him folk remedies for tuberculosis that trace back to the earliest years of the sanatorium movement: a quart of milk, cough syrup, soup: "good healthy stuff."

That we sense Ratso's sickness is tuberculosis is not surprising: the antituberculosis movement had drummed the disease into the public mind so persistently for three generations, and in so many different ways, that we absorb it automatically, without ever having to learn about it. Nor is it surprising that an awareness so systematically instilled should linger in the cultural air long after the disease itself had nearly vanished. What is surprising is the apparent reluctance to mention it, and the resulting aura it acquires as something mysterious, shameful, and obscene. In 1965 James Leo Herlihy treated the disease much as it might have been treated in 1870. It lurks, it threatens, it comes to symbolize death itself, and we all recognize it. But it can't be named.

You might attribute this to eccentricity, except that the sub-

sequent film does exactly the same thing. In doing so, moreover, it appealed to a mass audience. And *Midnight Cowboy*
is not alone. Between 1890 and 1950 America was flooded with
images of tuberculosis, and these images spilled out of the
medical arena into social policy, business; tuberculosis became
part of town life, a fixture in education, at times even a national
obsession. But from American literature—from the novel,
drama, poetry—it's strangely absent. It stimulated the imagination of the republic at large. Why, then, do writers appear
to ignore it?

For while American literature avoided the subject, at
roughly the same time European novelists virtually battened
on it. *The Magic Mountain* is the obvious example; for it consumption and the sanatorium were metaphorical vehicles not
merely for a study of life and death but for all European history, as the past teetered on the verge of the precipice from
which it was to plunge into World War I. And there were
others. Erich Maria Remarque returned to tuberculosis repeatedly; A. E. Ellis's 1958 novel *The Rack* exploited it in
detail.

The unassertiveness of consumption in American literature
might simply be laid down to chance if it weren't that the
peculiar difficulties it raised seemed to trouble writers themselves, and this is no better illustrated than in the case of Henry
James. *The Wings of the Dove* is, of course, the one indubitably
major American novel in which consumption plays a major
role. The heroine, Milly Theale, has it, dies of it; her sickness
is the pivot on which the elaborate plot of the whole book
turns.

Yet, as James himself somewhat embarrassedly noticed, that
center, in the course of the writing, simply disappeared. As
with *Midnight Cowboy*, sixty years later, tuberculosis is never
mentioned as such, never distinguished in the text by symptoms that would enable us to identify it. We absorb the diagnosis from the air, feeling the reverberation of James's very refusal to name it.

In his preface to the 1909 edition of the novel, James

bemusedly explores this paradox. "Why," he asks, "had one to look so straight in the face and so closely to cross-question that idea of making one's protagonist 'sick'?" Why avoid the crisis of a universally threatening and potentially fatal illness, so much the focus of so much human concern, and so obviously the stuff of drama? His initial answer is a plausible one: a novelist can't be preoccupied with dying as such. However sick the protagonist, it is the act of struggling *against* death that interests the writer, and not the relentless advance of the force that brings dissolution. If the novelist, then, is interested in life, he must inevitably favor the victim over the disease, and the disease itself must recede into the penumbra of the book.

A possible explanation, surely, yet James himself is plainly dissatisfied with it. After asserting that the real drama as he envisioned it was to be Milly's mortal struggle, he then admits that her peril leaves her "hanging so by a hair," and that the said hair, rather than suggesting the suspense of whether or not it will hold her up, hints rather that Milly must "fall somehow into some abysmal trap—this being, dramatically speaking, what such a situation most naturally implied and imposed." James has, in other words, made two rather slippery transitions, first from the disease itself to the struggles of the victim against it, second from her struggle against disease to her struggle against human opportunists who will try to exploit her weakness. He admits, as if with a sigh of relief, that this gave him the opening needed into his story—a welcome escape from the heroine by the act of imagining her persecutors, Kate Croy and Merton Densher. "It would be of the essence to create the predicament promptly and build it up solidly, so that it should have for us as much as possible its ominous air of awaiting her." Hence Kate Croy, who dominates the first third of the novel, and Merton Densher, her complaisant lover, the pair into whose clutches Milly falls.

Elliptically as always, James admits that Kate and Merton, healthy, devious, and selfish as they are, run away with the novel and that when Milly's great crisis comes, in Venice, he finds himself forced by the logic of his story not to render it through her eyes but theirs. Milly vanishes from her own great scene. "Heaven forbid, we say to ourselves during almost the whole Venetian climax, heaven forbid we should 'know' anything more of our ravaged sister than what Densher darkly pieces together. . . ."

For reasons James seems unable to formulate clearly, the linchpin of his story has to be suppressed, "imparting," as he phrases it, "to patches the value of presences." *"The Wings of the Dove,"* he confesses, "happens to offer the most striking example I may cite . . . of my regular failure to keep the appointed halves of my whole equal"; and confesses further on the author's half-amused despair at the "displacement of his general centre."

The Wings of the Dove is about tuberculosis; yet tuberculosis isn't there. James's model for Milly Theale was his beloved and much-idealized cousin, Mary Temple, who had died of consumption in 1870, more than thirty years before the writing of the novel. James had followed the course of her illness with anxious fascination. But the book has no night sweats, no hectic fever, no hemorrhages; not even Ratso Rizzo's cough, his complaints about colds or the flu. As Milly's end approaches, entirely offstage, Densher himself wonders at how completely the terrors of her illness have been expunged from the scene.

> . . . he had . . . , with everyone else, as he now felt, actively fostered suppressions which were in the direct interest of everyone's good manner, everyone's pity, everyone's really quite generous ideal. It was a conspiracy of silence, as the *cliché* went, to which no one had made an exception, the great smudge of mortality across the picture, the shadow of pain and horror, finding in no quarter a surface of spirit or of speech that consented to reflect it.

Yet despite this willful reticence, shared by the novel's characters and its creator, everyone knows what Milly's complaint is;

as she behaves, the literary critic F. O. Matthiessen remarked, "she can hardly be dying of anything except tuberculosis."

But how do we know? Because, indirectly and subliminally, James invokes all the spiritual paraphernalia of consumption, all the imagery it bore in the early nineteenth century, even as he suppresses the symptoms and the hope of cure that the antituberculosis movement was, even as he wrote, publicizing so assiduously. Milly is pale (the beleaguering villainess, Kate Croy, is dark), ethereal, spiritual; yet in spite of that or perhaps because of it, she's also powerfully erotic, even sexual, to a degree of explicitness unusual in James. Lord Mark, Densher's rival for Milly's hand, proposes to her thus:

> "You're not loved enough."
> "Enough for what, Lord Mark?"
> "Why, to get the full good of it."

It's plain in the context what "the full good of it" means, as is the innuendo when Kate agrees to spend a night with Densher in payment for his agreement to marry Milly for her money:

> "You'll come?"
> "I'll come."

Again, like Marguerite Gauthier in *The Lady of the Camellias* and Beth March in *Little Women,* Milly lives apparently normally, while the ravages of the disease imperceptibly advance within, communicating their progress only subliminally to observers at first, and expressing themselves as a heightened zest for life. Her physician, Sir Luke Strett, doses her with no drugs and prescribes no therapies except the intense enjoyment of life.

> "Shall I at any rate suffer?"
> "Not a bit."
> "And yet then live?"
> "My dear young lady," said her distinguished friend, "isn't to 'live' exactly what I'm trying to persuade you to take the trouble to do?"

Some Vague, Awful Thing

Milly floats through the novel in the metaphorical equivalent of a sanatorium, even though she never actually sets foot in one. James himself noted as a point of pride the clever recurrence of windows and balconies. Milly, like chasers of the cure, is ever looking down on a passing world from a high vantage. First and most notable is the scene in the Alps during which Susan Stringham, Milly's companion, unexpectedly comes upon her, perched on a precipice, "in a state of uplifted and unlimited possession. . . . She was looking down on the kingdoms of the earth, and though indeed that of itself might well go to the brain, it wouldn't be with a view of renouncing them. Was she choosing among them or did she want them all?"

Later, in Venice, the city of picturesque death, she ebbs away on an upper floor in her rented palazzo, approached by a grand staircase, viewing the world from a height half luxurious, half renunciatory:

The romance for her, yet once more, would be to sit there forever, through all her time, as in a fortress; and the idea became an image of never going down, of remaining aloft in the divine dustless air, where she would hear the plash of the water against stone. The great floor on which they moved was at an altitude, and this prompted the rueful fancy. "Ah not to go down—never, never to go down!" she strangely sighed to her friend.

Milly never will go down, as it happens, being fated to turn her face to the wall and die in the upper rooms of her palazzo, without marrying either of her two suitors. Not going down has multiple associations. The profane sexual one can't be discounted; still less can the sacred one. Milly, the dove of the title, doesn't, like the dove of the Bible, descend, but rather remains hovering on suspended wings. The dove descending is an image of pure spirit condescending to mix itself with the mire and complexity of material life; the very thing, for all Sir Luke's advice, Milly is tragically never able to do. James's names are never accidental; Sir Luke suggests the beloved

221

physician, St. Luke, in whose gospel the most explicit account of the descent of the dove at the baptism of Jesus occurs: Luke 3:21–23. And coexisting with the sacred and the profane dimensions of the image is a purely medical one—Milly is metaphorically the sanatorium inmate, perched on a magic mountain, looking down on the world from a vantage point above and removed.

If James's treatment emphasizes the mystic dimensions of the illness, shielding from our view the momentous events on the mountain peak (no more, after all, were the Jews allowed to see what went on between Moses and Yahweh on Sinai), it nonetheless still suggests, however elliptically, the clinical features of the disease and convinces us of it even when other characters avoid it. Kate and Merton Densher bring the possibility up only in order to deny it:

> "Is it a bad case of lungs?" he asked.
> Kate showed for a little as if she wished it might be. "Not lungs, I think. Isn't consumption, taken in time, now curable?"

We don't believe Kate partly because she's a liar, and she has something manifest to gain by this particular fib: she is trying to ease Densher into the thought that he might marry Milly, and at this point it's too early in her game to expose him to the crass fullness of the truth: that she'll inevitably die, leaving her fortune to Densher and the expectant Kate. Better to leave the illness unspecified, suggesting the hope of recovery without actually predicting it. But there is a better reason for disbelief in the ubiquitousness of the subliminal symptoms Milly herself has displayed—she is bathed in the aura of consumption even though its details are denied us.

All that said, why is James so adamant in his refusal to be explicit; why in fact is he antiexplicit, mentioning the disease only once, in the red herring of Kate's denial? James is of all novelists the master at indirection, screaming the very thing he appears to omit by placing a detail appropriately. In *The Ambassadors* we learn that a long-ambiguous relationship is in fact adulterous when the two conspirators drift into view in a rowboat, sighted by the novel's hero, Lambert Strether. Up to now, he's been wondering about the nature of their relation, but as they appear, the delicate, half-impalpable air of their behavior tells him what they are before he recognizes *who* they are:

> For two very happy persons he found himself straightway taking them—a young man in shirt sleeves, a young woman easy and fair, who had pulled pleasantly up from some other place, and, being acquainted with the neighborhood, had known what this particular retreat could offer them. The air quite thickened, at their approach, with further intimations; the intimation that they were expert, familiar, frequent—that this wouldn't at all events be the first time. They knew how to do it, he vaguely felt.

There can be no doubt about what this delicate network of airs and attitudes tells Strether, and tells him decisively: their relationship is no less clear to the reader because the language used to convey it is indirect.

There's something different about Milly's illness; it hovers outside the light of the text, looming and important, but never identified unambiguously, even by implication.

Why? James wrote the book, for one thing, under some pressure, composing the Venice chapters and Milly's death even as proofs for the first part of the book were arriving from the publisher. He was ill himself much of the time, and apart from having in Milly to recollect the still-painful death of Mary Temple, he was surrounded by other, more immediate reminders of mortality. In 1892 his sister Alice had died after years of invalidism, with Henry, unused to the bare face of death, watching horrified at her bedside.

> Toward the end, for about an hour, the breathing became a constant sort of smothered whistle in the lung. The pulse flickered, came and went, ceased and revived a little again, and then with all perceptible action of the heart, altogether ceased to be sensible for some time before breathing ceased.

In an odd turn of phrase in a letter to his brother William, he had written of Alice's "last breath," then crossed it out and substituted "the breath that was not succeeded by another." Alice died of breast cancer, which had perhaps spread to her lung toward the end, but James's act, even in the presence of death, of stepping back from it when he wrote of it, is suggestive.

Then he had, in 1894, been strongly affected by the death, in Venice, of Constance Fenimore Woolson, an old and close friend: she had jumped from an upper window of her house and died of the injuries, and it was in the wake of this event that he had jotted the first notes for *The Wings of the Dove*. So the atmosphere of the book was laden for James, not with a single painful memory but with several overlapping. Thrown in as well were other melancholy reminders: the recently published Balfour biography of Robert Louis Stevenson, the death of James's own pet wirehaired terrier.

All these might have prevented him from actualizing disease in his novel; but James had elsewhere proved able to fictionalize death, even Mary Temple's, even Constance Woolson's, without so oddly drawing back—witness *Daisy Miller* and "The Beast in the Jungle." James himself recognized the peculiarity of *The Wings of the Dove*. In writing *The Ambassadors*, he recalled, "I had absolute conviction and constant clearness to deal with; it had been a frank proposition, the whole bunch of data, installed on my premises like a monotony of fine weather." By contrast, *Wings* "was to worry me at moments by a sealing-up of its face—though without prejudice to its, again, of a sudden, fairly grimacing with expression."

Surely a part of the problem was his choice of *this* disease, consumption, weighted as it was with a burden of metaphor so immense that a writer could hardly invoke it without bringing down on himself a torrent of associations he had no wish to allude to. As Kate and Densher slyly remark in their short exchange, tuberculosis had, by 1901, roundly been pronounced curable: to bring it out too forthrightly would have forced James one way or another, to have dealt with sanatoriums, the Outdoor Life, surgery, blood, and perhaps even sputum cups; the book might, no doubt to James's horror, have blended in the public mind with the widely disseminated imagery of the anticonsumption crusade. Daisy Miller could die of Roman fever without forcing James on the one hand to describe the mosquito bite by which she would have contracted it, but also to be relatively frank about it without simultaneously encumbering his theme with a heavy burden of myth.

Nor was it only his culture that overdetermined the disease; it was James's own obsession with Mary Temple, magnified more by what she died of than the fact of her death. It's plain from his autobiographical memoir, *Notes of a Son and Brother*, that for James, Mary Temple either acquired from or gave to her tuberculosis the same spiritual refinement attached to it before the 1870s; her death just predated the new wave of thought about the disease, and it apparently fixed in James's mind an impression of spirituality that was to remain with him as late as 1914, when, long after *The Wings of the Dove*, he remembered his long-dead young cousin:

> It is always difficult for us after the fact not to see young things who were soon to be lost to us as already distinguished by their fate; this particular victim of it at all events might well have made the near witness ask within himself how her restlessness of spirit, the finest reckless impatience, was to be "met" by the common lot. . . . The charming, irresistible fact was that one had never seen a creature with such lightness of forms, a lightness all her own, so inconsequently grave at the core, or an asker of endless questions with such apparent lapses of care.

While his insistence on her vitality and her appetite for life somewhat attenuates her identity as a sylphlike, romantic consumptive maiden, the power of her spirit, the attraction she felt "to the prospect of the soul and the question of interests on *its* part that wouldn't be ignored," confirms her relation to

Beth March, Paul Dombey, and Marguerite Gauthier in her noble last days.

Still, all these attribute his reticence to personal factors, rather than to an endemic American reluctance to write in its imaginative literature about tuberculosis, when in fact James's silence in *The Wings of the Dove* is no more remarkable than James Leo Herlihy's in *Midnight Cowboy*.

Or, even more interesting, the movement from volubility to silence by Eugene O'Neill, who, in an early play, *The Straw*, tried to write about tuberculosis realistically, and from the authoritative though slippery ground of personal experience, but found the subject intractable and pronounced the play a failure. When he returned to it, in *Long Day's Journey Into Night*, he did so with the same gingerly touch one notes in other writers. He is an interesting case simply because his reticence was learned rather than apparently instinctive.

For O'Neill had had an early and decisive brush with tuberculosis; he was the only unquestionably major American writer who spent time as an inpatient at a sanatorium, and who afterward came to regard the experience as a formative part of his growth as a writer. He was struck in 1912, the fateful summer remembered in *Long Day's Journey.* He was ensconced at the Monte Cristo cottage, the family's New London summer home, working as a reporter for the local paper, the *Telegraph*, and churning out Dowsonesque verse with which he tried, often successfully, to impress girlfriends. That October he developed a bad cold, which lingered and worsened, leaving him with a persistent cough, fever, and night sweats; by November fluid had accumulated in his right lung and he began suffering occasional hemorrhages. Though his two physicians were slow to recognize the condition as tuberculosis, they were responsible men, a far cry from the quack James Tyrone engages for Edmund in *Long Day's Journey*. At least early in the course of the disease, James O'Neill's fabled stinginess, immortalized in James Tyrone, failed him: he even let the family hire Eugene a full-time live-in nurse, Olive Evans, who later remembered her patient as "a brilliant boy, but a little warped."

Only when it became evident that Eugene was consumptive
and in need of sanatorium treatment did James O'Neill's parsi-
mony emerge, in fact even exceeding James Tyrone's. He bul-
lied Eugene into the Fairfield County State Tuberculosis Sanatorium, a primitive encampment on the Otisville model,
located near New Haven, and serving mainly charity patients.
O'Neill had lived in the forecastle of a tramp steamer, in the
rat-infested warrens of Jimmy-the-Priest's three-dollar-a-
month boardinghouse (to which he later attributed his illness);
but he could not endure, for some reason, a charity hospital,
and stayed only two days. In a stormy confrontation with his
father in New York, O'Neill won his way and was sent to David
Lyman's Gaylord Farm Sanatorium in Wallingford; he arrived
there on Christmas Eve in 1912, in the middle of a blizzard.

Gaylord Farm had been in existence only eight years, but it
was already well known. Lyman was one of the founders of the
national association and became its president in 1918; his hospital embodied all the most advanced principles of the movement. It lay in an idyllic landscape, offered its patients pleasant
accommodations, good food, rest and exercise apportioned by
rule, and resolute optimism, which was generally justified by
results: 44 percent of Gaylord Farm's discharged patients were
well enough to earn their own livings five or more years after
they had left the hospital.

O'Neill flourished there, living proof of the assertion S. Adolphus Knopf was to make at Gaylord Farm's anniversary celebration a few years later—that a sanatorium was at base an
educational institution, with the patients as pupils and the
doctors as teachers. It was at Gaylord that O'Neill began, for
the first time, to turn his passion for writing into plays, and
there as well that he found, among both staff and patients, a
ready, appreciative, and no doubt to some extent captive audience. "It was at Gaylord," O'Neill later told the *Journal of the
Outdoor Life,*

that my mind got the chance to establish itself, to digest
and valuate the impressions of many past years in which

one experience had crowded on another with never a second's reflection. At Gaylord I really *thought about* my life for the first time, about past and future. Undoubtedly the inactivity forced upon me by the life forced me to mental activity, especially as I had always been high-strung and nervous temperamentally.

O'Neill made a confidant, even a mentor, of Lyman, keeping up a correspondence with him for years after his six months' stay at the hospital. "My blessings on the Farm 'spring eternal,' " he wrote Lyman in 1919, "and the recollections of my stay there are, and always will be, among the most pleasant of my memories." He made friends as well among the nurses, keeping in touch with one, Mary Clark, for years after his stay, and, in defiance of the rules, conducted a romance with a fellow patient, Catherine Mackay, a girl from a working-class Irish family in Waterbury.

This romance became the mainspring of O'Neill's 1921 play, *The Straw;* though largely ignored today, it is surely the most realistic portrayal of sanatorium life in American literature. Though the romance with Catherine Mackay provides it with its climax, the meat of the play is its careful reconstruction of sanatorium routine, with all its dramatic peaks and valleys, from arrival and adjustment to the good-byes between the lucky patient being released and the one still confined.

The plot of *The Straw* is creaky melodrama, though much of it does no more than recall O'Neill's stay at Gaylord Farm. Stephen Murray, aspiring writer and small-time reporter, arrives almost at the same time as Eileen Carmody, the hardworking Irish girl who, until stricken by consumption, has been the domestic mainstay for her stingy, drunken father (thus James O'Neill enters the play obliquely) and motherless siblings. A romance ensues, pursued lightly by the slightly ill Stephen, much more intensely by the apparently doomed Eileen. Stephen flourishes as Eileen languishes, losing weight week by week. Mrs. Turner, the practically omniscient matron of the sanatorium (and a portrait of Florence R. Burgess, a Gaylord Farm nurse), divines the reason and offers the approved sanatorium solution:

MRS. TURNER (looking at her keenly)
There is something upsetting you. You've something on
your mind that you can't tell me, is that it?

(EILEEN maintains a stubborn silence.)

MRS. TURNER (continuing)
But think—*can't* you tell me?
(with a kindly smile)
I'm used to other people's troubles . . . Can't you confide
in me, child?

(EILEEN drops her eyes but remains silent.
MRS. TURNER glances meaningfully over at
MURRAY who is watching them whenever he
thinks the matron is not aware of it—a note of
sharp rebuke in her voice.)

MRS. TURNER
I think I can guess your secret. You've let other notions
become more important to you than the idea of getting
well. And you've no excuse for it. After I had to warn you
a month ago, I expected *that* silliness to stop instantly.

Murray leaves the sanatorium, shocked by Eileen's midnight
confession that she has responded to his flirtation with a grand
passion, but returns in the last act. Eileen has, in his absence,
worsened to the point of death; in the play's climax, on Eileen's
sleeping porch, he vows altruistically to marry her.

She must marry me at once and I'll take her away—the
far West—any place Stanton thinks can help. . . . Oh Miss
Gilpin, don't you see? No half and half measures can help
us—help her. . . . But we'll win together. We can! We
must! There are things doctors can't value—can't know
the strength of! . . . You'll see! I'll make Eileen get well,
I tell you! Happiness will cure!

In reality O'Neill had not behaved so selflessly—Catherine
Mackay left Gaylord Farm a few months after O'Neill, never
heard from him again, and died within a year of her discharge.
But no doubt his reasons for rewriting truth had as much to do
with dramaturgy as self-exculpation—the events of sanatorium
life, charged as they were, demanded melodrama, even if that

entailed clumsiness. Sudden reversals, breathless arrivals, part-ings, deaths, weekly shocks (happy if your weight rose, nasty if it fell) were, after all, the bare realities of hospital existence; drama had to match itself to them.

O'Neill might have stood as an exception to the general unwillingness to treat tuberculosis as a visible entity, if he had left the theme upon finishing *The Straw*. But the play has been forgotten, mainly, perhaps, because of its clinical realism in the depiction of a forgotten and unpleasant phenomenon; also, paradoxically, because of its theatrics. Yet O'Neill went on to treat consumption in other plays, notably *Beyond the Horizon*, and—arguably his most successful drama—*Long Day's Journey Into Night*. And the irony here is that, precisely as the play succeeds, consumption retreats into background, into a dra-matic realm of repressions and reticences from which the emo-tional tension of the play arises.

O'Neill recalls the summer of 1912, and the family absorbing the shock of Edmund's disease. But all the impediments of the illness—the symptoms (except for a cough, heard most often offstage and witnessed by the audience only twice, once when his mother first appears in an addictive trance, and again in a final-act imbroglio with his father), the nurses, the consulting doctors—have been eliminated. Mary Tyrone, whose beloved father has died of the disease, superstitiously refuses even to name it and retreats into her morphine-induced stupor at least in part because she suspects Edmund may have it. The phalanx of competent medical personnel who in fact took care of O'Neill are reduced to a single quack who never actually ap-pears; even the phone call during which he gives James Ty-rone the diagnosis happens offstage.

Long Day's Journey draws much of its impact from denial; the temperature of the drama rises as more and more is em-phatically suppressed by the characters. Mary Tyrone's drug addiction and the refusal by her family to acknowledge its return is perhaps the most gripping example, but the central event, out of which the drama unfolds, is Edmund's tuberculo-sis. He denies it, James Tyrone denies it, Mary Tyrone hysterically and finally denies it. "The right way is to remember," Edmund says early in the play, echoing O'Neill's imperative in writing it. But the momentum is in favor of forgetting: "You mustn't remember!" Mary shouts at James Tyrone when he recalls her attempted suicide: "You mustn't humiliate me so!" And her passion for oblivion ultimately wins the day. At the climax, Edmund tries to tell her the truth; the disease tries to break into the play but fails.

EDMUND
Mama! It isn't a summer cold! I've got consumption!

> (For a second he seems to have broken through to her. She trembles and her expression becomes terrified. She calls distractedly, as if giving a command to herself.)

MARY
NO!

> (And instantly she is far away again.)

Therewith Mary drifts into another kind of memory—"What is it I'm looking for? I know it's something I lost"—less painful because less entangled with reality, a romantic vision of her childhood:

> Something I need terribly. I remember when I had it I was never lonely nor afraid. I can't have lost it forever, I would die if I thought that. Because then there would be no hope.

As she drags her wedding gown across the stage, the very emblem of dead hope, Mary echoes the ending of *The Straw*. There, O'Neill tried to pretend with his characters that hope can spring from a direct confrontation with mortality. But in the later play O'Neill sees a refusal to confront it as a well-spring of the drama; consumption becomes dramatic, the stuff of literature, by being repressed. If it might be said that Henry

James's obsession was usually to avoid the obvious, O'Neill's was generally to belabor it—his plays rarely understate their themes, are rarely remarkable for the terseness with which they are treated. Yet both concur in finding repression the most effective dramatic device for rendering tuberculosis.

This is not to suggest that either of them felt any such reluctance outside the realm of art. O'Neill spoke freely and affectionately, as we have seen, of his stay at Gaylord Farm; *The Straw* had committed him publicly to a quite accurate, even clinical rendering. James, in *Notes of a Son and Brother,* reproduced extensive quotations from some of Mary Temple's letters to his brother William, and these were perfectly matter-of-fact about the disease:

> The "it" of which I speak is my old enemy hemorrhage, of which I have had within the last week seven pretty big ones and several smaller, hardly worth mentioning. I don't know what has come over me—I can't stop them; but, as I said, I mean to try and beat them yet.

So we can't trace the peculiar note to repression on their part; it is simply that in American literature, without in any sense being ignored, tuberculosis has typically captured the imagination of writers for the effects *not* dealing with it directly can afford them.

The contrast with European literature is striking. Mann's *The Magic Mountain* was not just an attempt to capture a byway of human experience but the very essence of an epoch. The International Sanatorium Berghof at Davos may have been geographically removed from the great historical upheavals amidst which it appears to rest unaffected, but it's a fixed point from which they're all observed:

> Such institutions as the Berghof were a typical pre-war phenomenon. They were only possible in a capitalistic economy that was still functioning well and normally. Only under such a system was it possible for patients to remain there year after year at the family's expense. *The Magic Mountain* became the swan song of that form of

existence. Perhaps it is a general rule that epics descriptive of some particular phase of life tend to appear as it nears its end. The treatment of tuberculosis has entered upon a different phase today; and most of the Swiss sanatoria have become sports hotels.

Mann wrote these words in 1953, after the advent of antibiotics, but even at its first appearance in 1924, the novel expressed the full consciousness of its status as a chronicle of endings. It begins as the essentially passive hero, Hans Castorp, thoroughly a product of his place, his class, his time, climbs up to Davos in 1907 to visit his ailing cousin. Seven years later he descends into the middle of the great war, and the book closes as he dives into a foxhole to avoid an incoming shell.

The upward opening and downward closing movements of *The Magic Mountain* frame the magical seven years Hans Castorp spends at the sanatorium, apparently out of civilization's flow, yet watching it from the trance state the cure and the sanatorium lull him into. Though out of history, the sanatorium is a symbol of it; tuberculosis, while a disease that forces you into isolation from life, becomes a distillation of it. Unlike anything in American writing, *The Magic Mountain* is steeped in the lore of the cure; both the rituals and the rhythms of the sanatorium day and the sanatorium year. Though the Alpine institution ruled by its medical director, the Hofrat Behrens, has a definitively central European flavor, its methods were essentially the same as those so broadly advertised by the American antituberculosis crusade. The Outdoor Life ruled the cure at Davos as it did in Saranac, though with accommodations to European bourgeois demands: the Hofrat's cuisine is not merely hearty but Lucullan, and his medical attendance on his guests, as they are called, though authoritative, is gruffly deferential rather than paternal. But all the furniture of the routine is included: the thermometers, the sputum flasks, X rays, pneumothorax, thoracoplasty. Nor are they merely present; they are emphasized, and become vehicles for metaphor. On the one hand, Mann describes them all more realistically than anything one can find in American writing; on the other, he mines from them all the symbolic content they conceal.

The X ray, for instance. Having come up to Davos innocently for a rest, Hans finds himself suddenly and unaccountably beset by tubercular symptoms—the illusion of health vanishes, as, suddenly and shockingly, he finds himself among the invalids. He is summoned for his first X ray and fluoroscopy, and the procedure, as Mann describes it, is half pure science, half primitive magic. On the one hand, the Hofrat's blithe assurance makes it seem professional, technical, rational; but the flashing blue lights, the pulsation of machinery under the floor, and the milky glow of the fluoroscope screen suspended in the darkness touch the business with necromancy. "Can you see the hilus glands? Can you see the adhesions?" the Hofrat asks, as he watches his cousin Joachim being examined. "Look at the cavities here, that is where the toxins come from that fuddle him." But Hans notices something else, "like a bag, a strange, animal shape, darkly visible. . . . It expanded and contracted regularly, a little after the fashion of a swimming jelly-fish." The sight is Joachim's heart, and it provokes a spate of conflicting thoughts central to the novel, the collision between the new, rational regime of science and reason and an old, atavistic sense of magic and mortality, the last gasp of the Middle Ages as the modern age dawns.

Yet if the old mysteries are caught in the web of science and revealed, that web can also in turn be infiltrated and weakened by a recrudescence of mystery. Over the course of Hans Castorp's stay on the mountain, Dr. Krokowski, initially a proponent of psychoanalysis, becomes an avid researcher into the supernatural, a process that culminates in a séance in the former psychoanalytic consulting room. The vision, brought on by a phonograph recording of Valentine's Prayer from Gounod's *Faust*, is a return of the now-dead Joachim (he succumbs to tuberculosis about two thirds of the way through the novel); unutterably moving, it forms the climax of the story, a momentary reunion of past, present, and future that reflects in miniature the major theme of the whole book. Past and present in that, momentarily, the dead and the living meet; future in that Joachim appears in a uniform none of the participants recognize, since it is the gear of the coming war:

> But that was no proper uniform he wore. No colour, no decorations; it had a collar like a *litewka* jacket, and side pockets. Somewhere low down on the breast was a cross. His feet looked large, his legs very thin, they seemed to be bound or wound as for the business of sport more than war. And what was it, this headgear? It seemed as though Joachim had turned an army cook-pot upside-down on his head, and fastened it under his chin with a band.

The sight is an ironic message to Hans, who will shortly descend to fight in the war Joachim never lived to see; whether it is meant to be pitying or mocking isn't clear, though it overpowers Hans. "His throat contracted and a four- or five-fold sob went through and through him. 'Forgive me!' he whispered; then his eyes overflowed, he saw no more."

Mann had a lifelong obsession for turning apparently meaningless facts into symbols: business in *Buddenbrooks,* syphilis and music theory in *Doctor Faustus,* consumption and the sanatorium culture in *The Magic Mountain.* But though in the former cases his determination to find resonance in the dull or the scholarly is sometimes forced, it is not in the latter. Consumption opened a floodgate in his imagination that seems to have remained closed for American writers, and the echoes of shamanism that reverberate around the rituals of the Alpine hospital seem natural. Magical sevens abound—the seven years Hans spends on the mountain, the seven dining room tables each seating seven patients, the Walpurgisnacht celebration that occurs seven months into his stay, the digits of his room number thirty-four, which add up to seven; even, ironically, the surname of the book's indefatigable apostle of reason, skepticism, and humane science, Settembrini. Perhaps the most important conversation in the novel is a long debate, between Settembrini and Leo Naphta, the Jewish Jesuit, who, against Settembrini's rationalism, proposes a darker, more mystical, more antiquated, and more implacable philosophy. Both Naphta and Settembrini are tubercular, and cut off by their illness from the currents of the world they'd hoped to influence, but their very isolation clarifies the debate (without settling it). The disease, treated in full clinical detail, doesn't impede an exploration of other themes, but in fact encourages it.

Sickness, in Mann's perhaps pessimistic view, is not a sinister counterweight to life but identical with it, the metaphysical structure lying beneath. "What then was life?" the dim but earnest Hans Castorp asks himself at the beginning of his stay as a patient, when he forces himself, taken aback by his diagnosis, to study great issues.

> It was . . . a fever of matter, which accompanied the process of ceaseless decay and repair of albumen molecules that were too impossibly complicated, too impossibly ingenious in structure. . . . Disease was a perverse, a dissolute form of life. And life? Life itself? Was it perhaps only an infection, a sickening of matter? Was that which one might call the original procreation of matter only a disease, a growth produced by morbid stimulation of the immaterial?

Mann's fictional sanatorium, like America's real ones, was physically isolated in a mountain fastness, but it was intimately connected with the vital forces in the world from which it had seceded but of which it remained an accurate, distilled image. Hans, confined in the International Sanatorium Berghof, is visible, vital; Milly, curing in the upper reaches of her Venetian palazzo, simply vanishes from sight.

Mann's European imitators inherited his fascination, and his imaginative compulsion to endow consumption with explicit rather than merely hinted meaning. In fact, at times the details overwhelm the narrative, drowning out thematic undercurrents, so vehemently do they present themselves. A. E. Ellis's much-praised 1958 novel, *The Rack,* is in fact little more than a harrowingly detailed case history of its hero, Paul Davenant, a Cambridge student sent by government largesse to a sanatorium in the French Alps shortly after the close of World War II. He is tormented, like Hans Castorp, but less by metaphysical terrors than by the grinding horrors of his disease and the hard-hearted stinginess of the sanatorium, caring for its consignment of tubercular students and war veterans on a niggardly budget. Paul's story, told with grim, flat, unrelenting determination, is perhaps the most driven account ever written of the painful progress and the agonizing, catastrophic relapses characteristic of the disease. Paul's symptoms are described accurately and almost scientifically, without figuration, as if Ellis was determined not to distract the reader in any way from the pain of the facts.

The plot has the same contours as *The Magic Mountain*—it begins with the same railway ascent, describes the same socially diverse microcosm of invalids and doctors, and evokes the strange distortions of time that the cure visits upon its followers. Paul even has a romance, which, like Hans Castorp's, is initially conducted in French. But the similarity is casual; the story is a framework not for philosophizing but for painfully accurate reportage. Paul enters, receives a pneumothorax, but fails to improve because of a buildup of fluid in his pleural cavity, which necessitates what Dr. Vernet, his coolly, sardonically brutal physician, calls a *ponction sternale*. The procedure produces a crisis in Paul's cure and is described in terrifying detail.

> As the anaesthetizing needle penetrated Paul's side, it unnerved him. Then Dr. Vernet extracted it, and *Soeur* Miriam handed him a trochar-and-canulla, ten inches long. Paul tensed himself as Dr. Vernet plunged it adroitly between his ribs; it traversed the pleura and sank deeply.

The needle strikes blood; unfazed, Vernet merely lets it through a rubber tube into a large jar.

> At last the flow decreased to a trickle. Dr. Vernet disconnected the rubber tube and refitted the syringe to the

mouth of the canulla. Blood flowed once more; Dr. Vernet moved the canulla up and down in search of the last
drop. Paul gasped each time the end of the canulla
stabbed into his chest wall. *"Ça gratte un peu,"*
conceded Dr. Vernet, "but now it is finished." *Soeur*
Miriam handed Dr. Vernet the trochar, which she had
just sterilised over a spirit lamp, and Dr. Vernet replaced it in the canulla, and extracted the reassembled
instrument from Paul's side.

*"Mille trois cents c.c. de sang. Vous vous rendez
compte,"* declared *Soeur* Miriam grimly.

"Il ferait du bon veau. Vous l'avez bien saigné," said
Dr. Bruneau.

"What did he say?" demanded Paul.

"He said the best veal has the least blood. It is an
old French proverb much favoured in the butchery
trade. One says 'in the butchery trade,' or 'by the
butchery trade'? English prepositions I find very difficult."

Crisis follows crisis; recovered from this and many subsequent *ponctions sternales,* Paul succumbs to jaundice, and is
cut adrift when his sanatorium closes. He is dosed with antibiotics, newly available and injected directly into his chest cavity, but neither streptomycin nor PAS (a new antibiotic) do him
any good; nor do the doses of creosote that another physician
prescribes. He loses Michèle, his love, unsuccessfully tries to
kill himself with a dose of hoarded sleeping pills; and as the
novel closes he is facing the removal of one lung and the
knowledge that the other, hitherto sound, has been infected.
There is no interpretation, no gathering together of all this
suffering as a lesson of one kind or another, not even a hint that
it will end in death. The novel ends with the prospect that
improvement will follow relapse to be interrupted by further
relapse and still more drastic medical intervention, and that
the process will grind on indefinitely. Not only is tuberculosis
the disease not being suppressed by tuberculosis the metaphor; there is no metaphor whatever, and the illness stands by
itself as the medium of narrative.

The Rack was bought as a screenplay for an American film, but the movie, unsurprisingly, was never made; its imagination, or rather its dogged clinical literalism, runs against the sanitizing spirit of American imaginative renderings of the disease. Far more typical was the 1946 John Ford western, *My Darling Clementine.*

Doc Holliday, the dark and brooding *éminence grise* of the movie, has consumption, but we are never told so in the course of the film; Ford relies instead on the staple emblems of movie tuberculosis, a slight but nagging cough and a hovering air of doom. "Your health!" his friend-to-be Wyatt Earp toasts him at their first meeting in a Tombstone bar, and Doc responds with his first coughing fit, repeated at crucial junctures throughout the film. There are two heroes here, Wyatt and Doc; consumption tells us something about the contrast between them, and the contrast tells us something about the symbolic value so habitually attached to the disease during the twenties, thirties, and forties. Wyatt Earp, played by Henry Fonda, is the manifest hero, whose virtue is untroubled and clear, a direct and uncomplicatedly indignant reaction to the vices of others. His brother is murdered by the cattle-rustling Clanton gang; his revenge on them in the climactic gunfight at O.K. Corral is provoked by the Clantons themselves, not by any dark welling up of his own mixed motives but as a natural consequence of his duty as marshal of Tombstone.

But Doc Holliday, played by Victor Mature, is a damaged hero, noble but governed by darker and more mysterious forces of which his unspoken disease is an image, removing him as inexorably from direct scrutiny as Milly Theale's illness conceals her. We learn that he was once a successful Boston surgeon, who deserted his practice and his love (the Clementine of the title) to become the gambling czar of Tombstone; yet when Clementine tracks him down to ask why he's deserted her, he refuses to answer. Is it the doom his disease has inflicted on him, and his desertion a noble gesture, designed to spare his loved ones the sight of his decline and death? Or is it a sign of some mortal moral failing, of which the disease is only an image (or consequence), and of which his reputation as Tombstone's sinister baron is an expression?

Doc is drawn toward the good, noble, and pure—Wyatt, Clementine—yet held as well by something darker. When an itinerant actor passing through Tombstone is unable to recite Hamlet's "To be or not to be" speech, Doc moodily completes it for him, collapsing in a coughing fit at "Thus conscience doth make cowards of us all." Something in him attracts, indeed enthralls, the spotless Clementine, but when she appears in Tombstone he angrily orders her away, precipitating her into romance with the less tortured, healthy, and more fortunate Wyatt. Clues scattered throughout the film to the effect that Doc is in league with the vile Clantons take on a credibility dispelled only at the climax, when, the Clantons having challenged Wyatt to a gunfight, Doc sides with the latter. But even that final grand gesture, heroic though it is, is laced with failure. Before it Doc, overcoming his reluctance and his by-then-considerable drinking habit, performs emergency surgery on a gunshot victim, a temporary triumph ruined when the patient dies. And in the gunfight itself Doc's coughing nearly prevents him from firing and incapacitates him so that one of the Clantons is able to shoot him; he expires—though not before dispatching the offending Clanton—clutching a white handkerchief, as if to suggest that the death by shooting was only a quicker and more overt version of the mortality that had been eating away his vitals from the beginning of the story. Only Wyatt Earp, uncompromised and untainted, walks away from O.K. Corral to pursue his romance with Clementine; Doc Holliday perishes with the Clantons, though in the process he saves Wyatt.

If all this sounds more the stuff of hokum than myth, it omits the clarity, simplicity, and humor with which John Ford mounted it, qualities noticeably lacking in the overproduced 1957 remake, *Gunfight at the O.K. Corral,* directed by John Sturgis. In Ford's hands, the story, without pretending to subtlety, is nonetheless evocative, and Doc Holliday worthy to stand as a popular version of the consumptive hero as Milly

Theale is as a more arcane one. Great though the differences in their creators' ambitions are, the role consumption plays in both is strikingly similar. It heightens the drama by disappearing, refusing to be named yet insisting on being recognized. We know what it is and what it means, yet because it never emerges merely as a tissue of symptoms, it suggests other mysteries and other horrors, mental and moral as well as spiritual. Sometimes the secret seems angelic, as with Milly Theale; sometimes demonic, as in the tortured relations of Eugene O'Neill's Tyrones; sometimes unfathomable, as with Doc Holliday. But it is never the challenging but curable disease of the antituberculosis movement, never the manageable nemesis to be conquered by fresh air, rest, method, and optimism. It lurks, it hovers; both the characters and the audience know what it is; but none names it.

This was true even when Americans adapted more explicit European stories for the domestic market. Erich Maria Remarque's *Drei Kameraden,* translated into English in 1937 as *Three Comrades,* is, for all its romanticism, a realistic portrayal of its heroine's galloping consumption, which bursts out at a seaside holiday with her lover and ends, grimly, at a sanatorium. The novel closes with the narrator, her lover, numbed, spending a night with her corpse:

> Then I washed the blood from her. I was like wood. She grew cold. I laid her in my bed and covered her with the bedclothes. I sat beside her and could not think. I sat on the chair and stared at her. The dog came in and sat with me. I watched her face alter. I could do nothing but sit vacantly and watch her. Then morning came and it was she no longer.

In 1938 *Three Comrades* was made into a movie, produced by Joseph Mankiewicz and with a screenplay by F. Scott Fitzgerald (of all the scripts Fitzgerald worked on during his bilious Hollywood period, this was the only one ever to be produced, though Fitzgerald was forced to accept a collaborator,

E. E. Paramore), and while the resulting movie is more explicit than the run of Hollywood treatments—there are sanatorium scenes, for example—it is far less so than Remarque's novel. Pat, the heroine, has a hemorrhage (not shown directly, but hinted at in a dark stain on a towel by her head), but tuberculosis is never mentioned by name. The death scene, unsurprisingly, is truncated and romanticized.

> PAT (very low)
> It's all right—it's hard to die—but I'm quite full of love—like a bee is full of honey when it comes back to the hive in the evening.
>
> (On these words, before her eyes close in death, we—)
>
> FADE OUT

This scene is followed by the conclusion: as Pat's surviving lover, Bobby, fights Nazis in the city streets, he is joined by the shadowy figure of Pat, who walks beside him "toward whatever lies ahead." Sentiment may have been the main motive behind the changes Fitzgerald and Mankiewicz made in the story, but their declinicalizing of consumption is an American commonplace.

Why? Europe had no antituberculosis movement as widespread and as vastly publicized as America's. Perhaps our pamphlets, advertisements, billboards, lectures, radio programs, direct mail campaigns, and propaganda films simply stole tuberculosis from literature. So frenetic was the public-benefit image making that it may simply have overwhelmed any private creative impulse; S. Adolphus Knopf, Hermann Biggs, and their colleagues may have staked such a domineering claim to the picturing of consumption that they frightened off the novelists and the playwrights. And perhaps this was more than mere imperialism in the public health fraternity; perhaps the public wanted its image of tuberculosis managed by a collegial body of professional activists rather than literary mavericks and creative loose guns. Concord, in remaking the dead Thoreau in its reassuring if erroneous image of the disease, had long before illustrated that the public has a stake in constructing the way we all look at something as important as the most mortal of all diseases; the process of defining it is not left to individuals. Perhaps, then, the absence of the disease from American literature (or rather the constant presence never explicitly acknowledged) may simply be a tribute to the effectiveness of the antituberculosis movement, which had made the disease a public thing, wrenched it away from the individual, and made it a collective property and a collective obsession. A novelist might, then, be no more likely to describe the specifics of it than he would the specifics of the highway system or the telephone network. All were complex, all worth attention, but all in themselves too publicly fixed to be remade by the writer's imagination.

Yet, again, perhaps the elliptical literary response to consumption is as much a criticism as an act of deference. The public campaign had labored mightily to demystify it, transforming it from a dark terror into a serious but meetable challenge. The cure, in the crusade's propaganda at least, ceased to be a hazardous personal quest ridden by nightmare and became a jolly group hobby. A century of scientific progress had transformed the disease in the public mind from an inscrutable visitation into a clearly defined syndrome caused by a single microbe; by the twenties and thirties, patients were, in their reminiscences and their sanatorium magazines, chummily calling the bacilli "bugs"; they'd been demythologized, or rather remythologized as pesky but manageable. Perhaps literature was restoring the balance, reminding us that the darkness so confidently dispelled by the crusade in fact remained. Isabel Smith had kept her Trouble Book for the black thoughts that couldn't be uttered and the terrible questions that couldn't be asked—even as, in the public world of the sanatorium, among doctors, nurses, and fellow patients, she exuded confidence. Yet the troubles couldn't be entirely forgotten; something had to attest to their continuing though suppressed existence. Perhaps it was this need that the novelists, playwrights, and filmmakers were answering. Wyatt Earp was the kind of man Knopf would have praised (in *Gunfight at the O.K. Corral* he gruffly suggests that Doc check himself into a hospital near Denver). Doc Holliday, on the other hand, was better suited to the darknesses and ambiguities of literature.

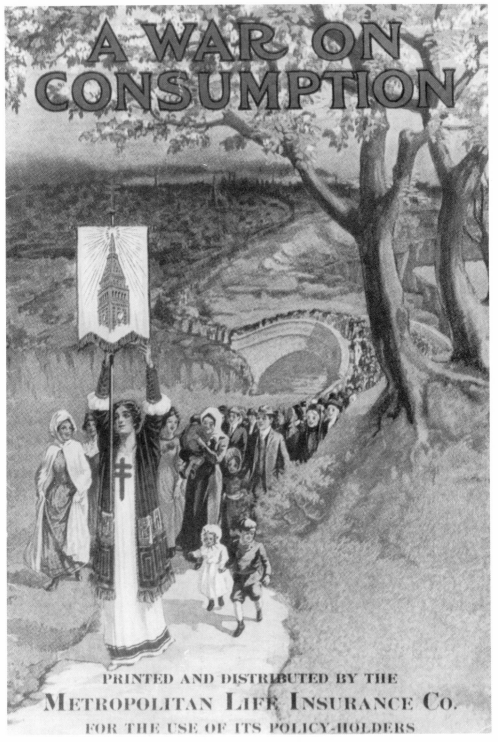

A WAR ON CONSUMPTION

PRINTED AND DISTRIBUTED BY THE
METROPOLITAN LIFE INSURANCE Co.
FOR THE USE OF ITS POLICY-HOLDERS

Hygeia delivering the masses: cover illustration from the Metropolitan Life
Insurance Company's 1915 pamphlet, *A War on Consumption*. *(Courtesy of the
Metropolitan Life Insurance Company Archives)*

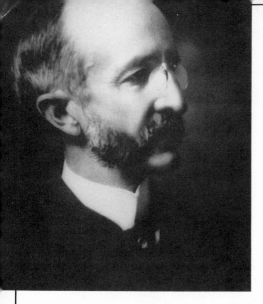

Edward Livingston Trudeau, M.D., American pioneer of the sanatorium movement and leader, during its early years, of the anti-tuberculosis crusade. *(Courtesy of the Trudeau Institute Biomedical Research Laboratory, Saranac Lake, New York)*

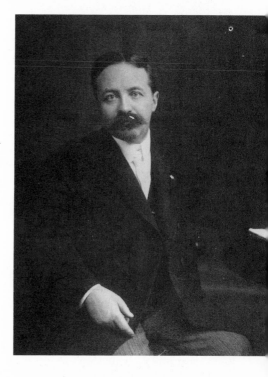

S. Adolphus Knopf, M.D., author of the prize-winning *Tuberculosis as a Disease of the Masses and How to Combat It* and tireless public advocate for the tubercular. *(Courtesy of the Trudeau Institute Biomedical Research Laboratory, Saranac Lake, New York)*

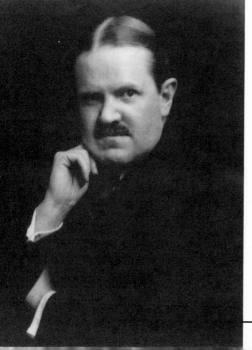

Saranac Lake physician, Lawrason Brown, M.D., devised and refined the detailed sanatorium regimen later adopted by the national movement. *(Courtesy of the Trudeau Institute Biomedical Research Laboratory, Saranac Lake, New York)*

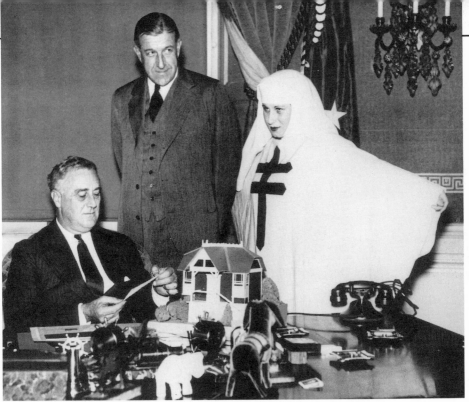

Hygeia presents F.D.R. with a model of the Little Red, America's first sanatorium cottage, while Dr. Francis B. Trudeau looks on. *(Courtesy of the Trudeau Institute Biomedical Research Laboratory, Saranac Lake, New York)*

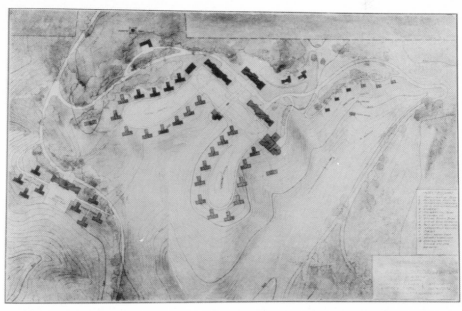

Site plan for the Georgia State Sanatorium at Alto. Structures outlining the brows of the twin hills and suggesting lungs are the rest cottages. The Administration Building is the large edifice at the upper right. Note the hospital for black patients in the lower left-hand corner. *(From Thomas S. Carrington,* Tuberculosis Hospital and Sanatorium Construction, *1911)*

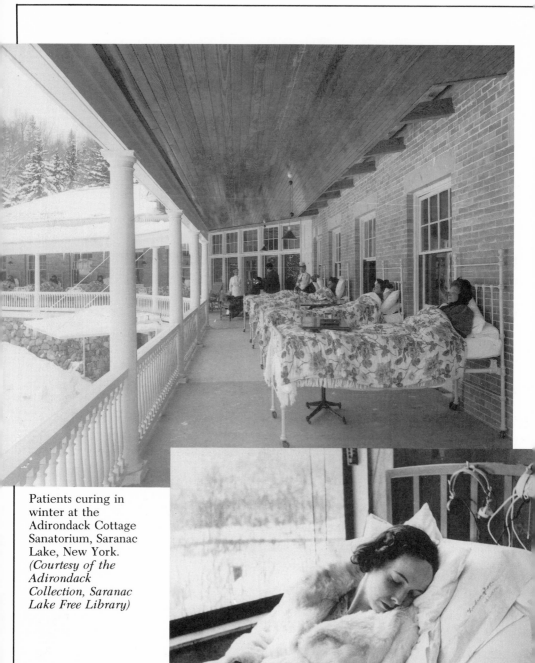

Patients curing in
winter at the
Adirondack Cottage
Sanatorium, Saranac
Lake, New York.
*(Courtesy of the
Adirondack
Collection, Saranac
Lake Free Library)*

Isabel Smith, asleep in her room at the Trudeau Sanatorium's
Ludington Infirmary, 1937. *(Photograph by Alfred Eisenstaedt,
courtesy of* Life *magazine © Time Inc.)*

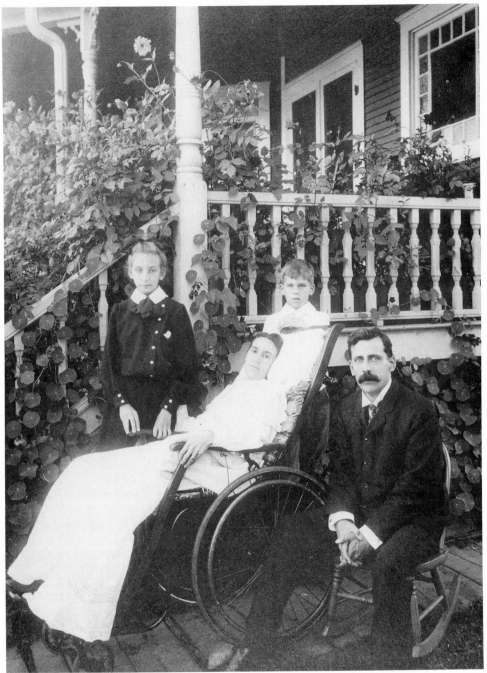

A family, in Saranac Lake for the cure, posed before the Blauvelt Cottage on Helen Hill, early 1900's. *(Courtesy of the Adirondack Collection, Saranac Lake Free Library)*

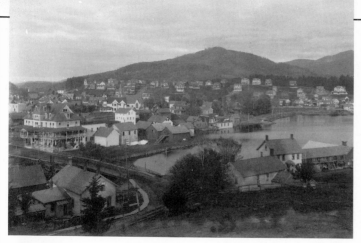

Saranac Lake, New York, looking northeast across Lake Flower, circa 1905. The large building at the left is the Riverside Inn, usually the first stop for healthseekers arriving in the village. *(Courtesy of the Adirondack Collection, Saranac Lake Free Library)*

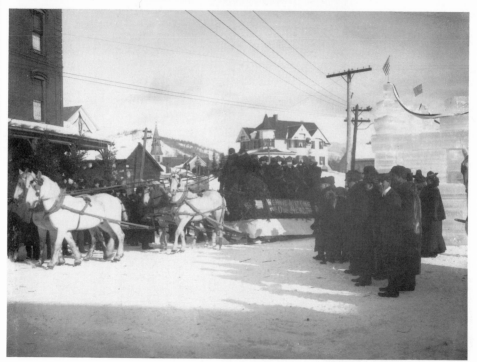

Mid-winter carnival, Saranac Lake, early twentieth century. The Ice Palace is at the right, a horse-drawn float, bearing healthseekers, at the left, blazoned WE HAVE JUST COME FOR OUR HEALTH. *(Courtesy of the Adirondack Collection, Saranac Lake Free Library)*

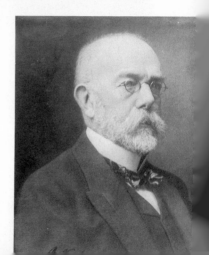

Robert Koch, pioneer bacteriologist, in 1910. Koch had discovered the tubercle bacillus in 1882, and promoted a disastrous "cure," Koch's Lymph, in 1890. *(Courtesy of the New York Academy of Medicine Library)*

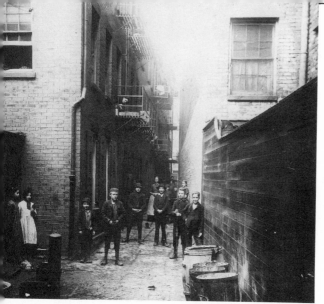

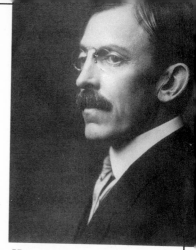

Back tenements behind number 32 Cherry Street, New York City, in the late 1880s, vicinity of the Lung Block, the city neighborhood most infamous for its death rate from tuberculosis. *(Photograph by Richard Hoe Lawrence, courtesy of The New-York Historical Society, New York City)*

Hermann M. Biggs, M.D., New York City, later state health commissioner, was a leading advocate, beginning in the 1890s, of public health law as a weapon against the spread of consumption. *(Courtesy of the Trudeau Institute Biomedical Research Laboratory, Saranac Lake, New York)*

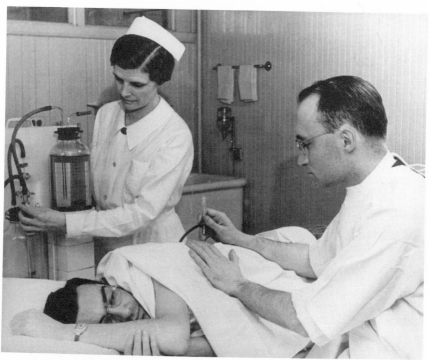

A patient receiving artificial pneumothorax treatment at the Trudeau Sanatorium, 1937. *(Photograph by Alfred Eisenstaedt, courtesy of* Life *magazine ©* Time Inc.)

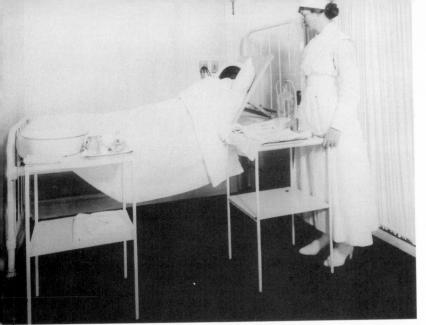

Nurse and patient at the Trudeau Sanatorium, circa 1930. *(Courtesy of the Trudeau Institute Biomedical Research Laboratory, Saranac Lake, New York)*

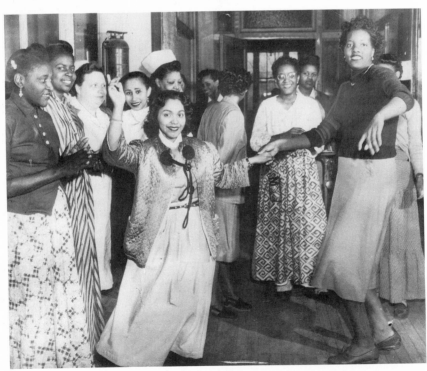

Patients dancing at the Sea View Sanatorium, Staten Island, New York, 1953. "A few months ago," according to the caption circulated with this newsphoto, "only the sound of TB victims coughing their lives away could be heard here." The startling improvement followed the introduction at Sea View of iproniazid, a highly stimulative variant of the new antibiotic isoniazid. *(Courtesy of AP/ Wide World Photos)*

9

"The Haunted Hospital":
Antibiotics and the Closing of the Sanatoriums

For miles around you could see it. . . . You'd drive up a
long, winding hill, overgrown with bushes, and come to
a chain link fence. And everybody always thought,
whatever the disease was—and none of us knew—you'd
get it if you went inside. We called it "The Haunted
Hospital" . . .

—MARSHALL WATSON, RECALLING
A VISIT TO AN ABANDONED
KANSAS CITY SANATORIUM IN
THE MID-1960s

41 Park Ave.
Saranac Lake, N.Y.
June 11, 1952

His Excellency Governor Thomas Dewey

Dear Governor Dewey,

  *Wrote a letter May 10, 1952 to you concerning patients
for our local sanatorium cottages. Tubercular county patients from Manhattan N.Y.C., or Albany . . . just don't
have the means of paying there [sic] own way and our
rates are more reasonable than in hospitals. . . . Why not
send some to our local cottages as we all need help badly?*
  *I do hope you will read this letter with interest and not
consider it just another letter as we are equipped to care
for tubercular patients and would appreciate . . . not charity but work. Governor Dewey, mostly all the local san.
folks own there [sic] cottages which [are] very hard for us
to maintain with taxes so high without help. . . . I am
certain you can help us.*
  *May I also add this is a Republican town and our men
and women work very hard for the party being that the*

party is in control in Albany. Nothing should stop you, Governor Dewey, from aiding us. . . .

Sincerely,

MRS. ISABEL SHANNON

Sporck and Shannon Cottage

When Mrs. Shannon wrote her desperate appeal, the cure was languishing. Streptomycin, the first antibiotic effective against tuberculosis, had been discovered in 1944 and became a routine though not wholly satisfactory part of treatment by 1947. And worse was to follow, though Mrs. Shannon could not have known it; in January of 1952 two pharmaceutical companies, Squibb and Hoffmann–La Roche, had announced the production of a new, synthetic antibiotic, isoniazid, which, upon testing, was to prove the decisive component in the victory over consumption and lead, in no short time, to the end of the sanatorium era.

Yet the malaise her letter reflects was not, at least not entirely, the product of the new revolution in chemotherapy, for streptomycin had not yet replaced either surgery or long-term bed rest as the principal treatment plan, and there were still large numbers of consumptives, though cancer had edged out tuberculosis as a cause of death in the 1930s, as heart disease had done in the late 1800s. Rather, the decline in tuberculosis that was now beginning to cause such distress in the economy of the cure had begun, paradoxically, before the War on Consumption was even a vision, let alone a reality. Statistics for the nineteenth century are at best unreliable, since before Robert Koch tuberculosis could not definitively be diagnosed; other diseases might be mistaken for it. But as best most experts can judge, mortality from consumption peaked, in both the United States and Europe, around 1840, at least thirty years before the shift in attitudes that changed it in the public mind from a spiritually uplifting affliction to a degrading but conquerable enemy. In that sense, the antituberculosis crusade, whatever its methods, was foredoomed to success, arrayed as it was against an already weakening and retreating foe. By 1900–1904, perhaps the first date for which absolutely reliable statistics exist, tuberculosis in the United States was causing 184.8 deaths per 100,000 people per year. This represented roughly 11 percent of all deaths at the time. Though tuberculosis was less mortal than cardiovascular disease, it was three times more often a cause of fatality than cancer. But within twenty years, mortality from tuberculosis was to decrease by half, to 97.1 per 100,000 in the 1920–24 period, perhaps the peak of the sanatorium era. By 1944, still before the introduction of streptomycin, the death rate had halved again, to 43.4 per 100,000, and the White Plague had been passed by influenza and pneumonia as a factor in mortality.

Saranac Lake had begun to notice the inevitable effect on its economy in the 1930s, though of course the longer-term cause of the decline was at least temporarily masked by the immediate crises of the Depression. But the ill stopped arriving in ever-increasing numbers; the town's population, hitherto burgeoning, stagnated; and business fell off. "We have a bare existence as is in this part of the country," Mrs. Shannon had written in an earlier letter to Governor Dewey that had disappeared into the caverns of the state bureaucracy, and it was fated to become barer. Streptomycin hastened the end; isoniazid, in general use by 1953, assured it. By 1967 tuberculosis was causing only fourteen new cases and 4.1 deaths per 100,000 per year. From the time reliable record keeping began to be possible, around 1900, both new cases of tuberculosis and deaths from it had been declining at a rate of from 4 to 6 percent a year; and with the introduction of antibiotics, the falloff rate doubled.

How did it come about, this triumph over a dreaded disease? Antibiotics are the easy answer, because they were a brand-new factor in the 1940s, and their effects were easily measurable, both in the patients who took them and, subsequently, in the morbidity and mortality statistics; scientists can also explain, though not as completely as they would like, how antibiotics affect the tubercle bacillus. But it's a thornier matter to find reasons for the major declines that preceded antibiotics; experts have never agreed on a single cause, and there is no firm, empirically grounded consensus even on a possible combination of causes. Perhaps tuberculosis waned because of the advent of the sanatorium rest cure and the new surgical techniques devised as supplements to it in the twenties and thirties, though both remained controversial, and their effectiveness was never conclusively demonstrated. Or perhaps the improvement came from better living conditions—better housing, better food, more careful and more frequent health screening—though the decline in tuberculosis morbidity and mortality persisted unabated through a severe decline in living standards during the Depression. Again, perhaps natural selection performed the miracle, as, over the generations, the susceptible were culled from the gene pool and the resistant survived to reproduce. Or perhaps the disease was simply following a cycle of its own; as *mycobacterium tuberculosis humanis* evolved, perhaps it changed its habits and became less virulent. We had no way of knowing its intimate secrets, after all, until 1882.

Whatever the reasons, by 1920 the situation was both immensely encouraging and agonizingly frustrating: the economic crisis to be brought on by the final victory was still nearly a half century away. On the one hand, great strides had been made: patients were being cared for and, at least in some cases, apparently cured; the well were being protected from the sick and being effectively urged to protect themselves from the consequences of their own bad health habits. Urban conditions favorable to the spread of disease had been attacked if not eliminated. Yet, despite a significant decline in deaths from consumption, the disease remained potent, and a knockout triumph over it remained elusive. This was an irritant to physicians and scientists as well as a continuing threat to the public, for, as we have seen, the medical fraternity had arrived at only an uneasy and unstable truce in the treatment of the disease. Bacteriology, apparently the wave of the future, had scored a major triumph with Koch in 1882, and Abraham

Flexner had, with the tacit consent of the medical profession, made its laboratory methods the cornerstone of reform in medical education. Yet the early optimism had struck an iceberg in the disaster with Koch's lymph in 1890, and now, thirty years later, though bacteriological research had accumulated a large body of knowledge about the tubercle bacillus and its behavior in the human host, the triumphant therapy Koch had dared to envision as a consequence of his discovery remained unfound. The sanatorium regimen, as invented by Brehmer and Dettweiler, Americanized by Trudeau, and elaborated by Lawrason Brown and his contemporaries, could claim some plausible success; but it wasn't so much science as art and folklore, adapted as far as possible to take advantage of what science had revealed about the disease process. In 1920 the average sanatorium was closer to a summer camp or a health resort than it was to a modern hospital, and the medical director presided over it more as a father figure and a teacher than as a dispenser of effective medicines or a performer of surgery. His presence reassured the patients and guaranteed that the cure would proceed along lines consistent with emerging knowledge about the disease; through X rays, temperature charts, weigh-ins, physical examinations, and sputum analysis, he could tell them how they were progressing. But he could do no more, and the literature of the antituberculosis movement of the time expected no more.

An unsatisfactory situation for an ambitious profession of which so much was expected. Doctors were thus not content with the status quo; it reeked of the era when the doctor was, even where he earned respect, an artisan, at a time when he was aspiring to be a scientist with an armory of surefire technically elaborate therapies. In 1917, partly to consolidate and disseminate rapidly accumulating knowledge but also to root the crusade firmly in science, the national association founded the *American Review of Tuberculosis*. In its early years the journal devoted as many of its pages to studies of the sociology of tuberculosis as it did to purely scientific studies, and even technical articles were often written as essays, as much exercises in style as in the experimental method: the physicians who wrote them had not yet abandoned their heritage as cultured gentlemen in favor of their future as technocrats. But as time went on, the *Review* became steadily more devoted to hard science; essays gave way to bald presentations of data and experimental results; individual authors who paid attention to their prose gave way to teams of researchers who wrote as featurelessly as possible. This was, perhaps, the inevitable result of the stasis that, in 1917, seemed, for all the minor advances, to have afflicted bacteriological study. For all its optimism, the inaugural issue of the *Review* carried an editorial that quietly acknowledged the problem:

> The 1880s was the decade of the bacillus, the 1890s that of tuberculin [the newly coined term for Koch's lymph], while the last decade has been noteworthy because the wheat of the two former eras has been separated from the chaff, and has been brought into harmony and coordination.

But consolidation was not enough; it was only the starting point for a more concerted scientific effort not only to understand the bacillus but to study its effects on the invalid:

> We no longer look at the bacillus as the sole factor in the production of the disease tuberculosis. We no longer regard tuberculin either as a cure-all or as anathema. We have learned that besides a seed tuberculosis requires a soil. . . . We now appreciate that we must study not only the offending microorganism but also the smitten host.

More study, in other words, not only of the microbe but of the victim, in the hope that hitherto-elusive techniques might emerge by which the disease process could be stopped or reversed. Koch's lymph, or tuberculin, had so far proved worse than useless as a cure (though hopeful experiments persisted), but by 1908 it had gained a new and vital function as a diagnostic tool. Injected under the skin, it caused a rapid and unmistakable inflammation in anyone who had been exposed to the disease; this rapidly established that a large majority of humans had been at one time or another invaded by *mycobacterium tuberculosis humanis.* Koch's own violent reaction to the injection of lymph he gave himself as an experiment revealed that he was among the number, though of course he failed to realize it at the time. Perhaps research would show why, in most people, the disease remained subclinical and why, among the unlucky few, it raged on unchecked. The answers, if they could be found, might suggest techniques by which the ill could be armed artificially against the disease as the well were naturally.

The quest for such techniques soon split into two wings, one surgical, one bacteriological. The twenties and thirties were an era in which surgery enjoyed a particularly high reputation, while bacteriological studies, at least with regard to consumption, languished, and in the two decades following the First World War, tuberculosis patients were far more likely to undergo surgery than experimental chemotherapy. Research with antibiotics proceeded slowly and fitfully, but surgical techniques were available even at the beginning of the sanatorium era, though it took some time for them to establish themselves as part of the cure.

In the 1880s, for instance, Carlo Forlanini, an Italian surgeon, began reporting favorable outcomes from artificial pneumothorax. If rest fostered improvement in the diseased lung, it followed, at least in theory, that healing would progress more rapidly still if the lung were, as far as possible, completely immobilized by allowing air to enter the intrapleural space (later it was argued that collapse deprived the tubercle bacilli of needed oxygen). In 1892 Forlanini described the procedure and offered a clinical rationale for it.

> The lung . . . becomes consumptive because, differently from all the other viscera, it is in an unceasing motion of expansion and reduction. . . . The phthisogenic process must terminate in the lung which is immobilized by pneumothorax.

In the United States the procedure found a characteristically feistier advocate in James Benjamin Murphy, a surgeon aggressive in touting his craft and eager to see it make its mark on the therapy of consumption. In 1898 he delivered an Oration on Surgery at the annual meeting of the American Medical Association. What, he demanded, could physicians show for all their bacteriological advances in the last decade? With the exception of "a thorough knowledge of its etiology and pathology," he responded, "comparatively nothing." His solution was brisk and simple: "allow the wall of the [tubercular] abscess to collapse, to empty thoroughly, and it will heal, as other abscesses of the same character."

At first, artificial pneumothorax was slow to win adherents, but the International Congress of Tuberculosis endorsed it formally at Rome in 1912, and thereafter it spread rapidly. World War I produced an alarming upsurge in tuberculosis in Europe, and a corresponding demand for therapy, which the surgeons rushed to fill. (Perhaps the very butchery of the war prepared the public to accept this relatively invasive and somewhat painful procedure the more readily.) By the 1920s it was common; by the 1930s it had spread to America and become routine. In 1937 between 50 and 80 percent of the patients at major American sanatoriums were undergoing it, though it remained a subject of contention among physicians and was much less frequent at smaller hospitals—in a thorough 1935 study published in the *American Review of Tuberculosis* the authors reported that, nationwide, an average of 10 percent of all tuberculosis patients embarked on a course of pneumothorax. It was not usually a one-time thing. Murphy had optimistically hoped that a single total collapse of the affected lung would produce a cure, but Forlanini argued instead for a long-sustained course of partial collapses, renewed periodically, and his view prevailed. Once you began pneumothorax you lived with it—and its related annoyances—for months, often for years.

Like everything else in the sanatorium, it became a ritual. It had a nickname—"pneumo" or "gas" (for the air introduced between the lung and the chest wall)—and it marked an intermediate stage of the cure, after the patient had undergone his gestatory period of bed rest and clinical evaluation. It could be performed at the bedside and didn't hurt much; after the first session it was often done without anesthetic. Typically the patient lay on his stomach with his arm over his head, as the easiest entry into the chest cavity was between the ribs in the area of his armpit. Then the pneumothorax machine was wheeled up, a memorable device consisting, usually, of two bottles partly filled with fluid (a mixture of water and antiseptic, dyed for easy visibility) and joined by a rubber tube. One of the bottles was partly filled with air and calibrated; a tube ran from the air chamber to a needle. If the fluid-filled bottle was raised, water would flow into the other bottle, forcing air out of the top, through the tube and needle, and into the intrapleural space. The calibrations allowed a careful monitoring of the amount of air being injected.

Betty MacDonald recalled her first experience with the procedure:

> I felt the prick of the hypodermic needle, just under my left breast, then an odd sensation as though he were trying to push me off the table [the physician was forcing the pneumothorax needle through the muscle], then a crunchy feeling and a stab of pain [as the needle punctured the sensitive pleura]. "There now," the Medical Director said, as he attached the end of what looked like a steel knitting needle to a small rubber hose connected to two gallon fruit jars partially filled with a clear amber fluid. The nurse put one jar higher than the other and I waited frantically for my breathing to stop and suffocation to start. There was no sensation of any kind for a few minutes then I had a pulling, tight feeling up around my neck and shoulder. The doctor said, "I guess that's enough for today," took the needle out, slapped a bandage on me and I got down from the table, dizzy with relief.

That, normally, was that, until, after a week or two, the air dissipated and the procedure had to be repeated in order to maintain the collapse.

This could lead to accidents and complications. The doctor could tell where the needle was only by touch, and that could be deceptive—it might lodge accidentally in the thickness of the pleura itself, in a pulmonary blood vessel (in which case blood would spurt up through the needle and into the tube), or even, disastrously, in the lung. If, somehow, a bolus of air from the apparatus got into the circulatory system, it might strike the brain and cause convulsions, blindness, or paralysis. And in many patients a collapse couldn't be effectively produced, since the section of the pleura lining the inside of the chest wall frequently became attached at one or more points to the section covering the outside of the lung, and the resulting adhesions, as they were called, pulled the lung along with the chest wall as the latter expanded and contracted, no matter how much air was forced into the intrapleural space. To that complication, the surgeons devised solutions. The most usual was called intrapleural pneumolysis (the terminology got more complicated as the procedures did). The surgeon cut two holes in the chest wall, one for a thoracoscope, the other for a cauterizing instrument. Using the thoracoscope, he searched for adhesions, burning them away with the cauterizing instrument when he encountered them and, he hoped, freeing the lung from surrounding tissue in order to allow a successful collapse. This operation, too, spread throughout sanatoriums in the United States and became a standard accompaniment to pneumothorax in the 1930s.

Nor was it the only one. Surgeons, vying for efficiency and renown, devised an exotic variety of techniques for immobilizing the lungs, each of which had its brief fashion. In oleothorax you filled the chest cavity with oil instead of air. In *extra*pleural pneumolysis, the surgeon stripped the lung and *both* pleural layers away from the rib cage and packed the resulting space either with spare abdominal fat or with wax. In pneumoperitoneum, air was injected into the abdominal cavity, and the consequent elevation of the diaphragm compressed the lung. If the surgeon was disposed to meddle with the nervous system instead of the muscles and bones, he would launch an attack on the phrenic nerve, which controlled the diaphragm. It could be crushed with forceps, or, in a rather more harrowing procedure, plucked out of the diaphragm and reeled up through the chest like a loose thread being drawn out of cloth. In either case the diaphragm, partly paralyzed, immobilized the lung above. Those favoring simple solutions might recommend a resection, or removal of the diseased part of the lung.

But the king of operations, reserved for cases where other techniques failed to produce a satisfactory collapse, was thoracoplasty. Devised by Ludolph Brauer of Marburg and refined by two other German surgeons, Max Wilms and Ernst Ferdinand Sauerbruch, it was the most radical and disfiguring of all the available techniques. In it the surgeon simply removed the ribs, sometimes eleven, sometimes only nine. At first the ribs were simply broken away from the spine and discarded, but mortality was so high that surgeons began removing only those sections of the ribs near the vertebrae and left the ventral segments floating more or less free in the musculature of the front of the patient's chest. They took out only the bone, leaving the periosteum, or bone-covering membrane, which, in time, generated cartilagelike pseudo-ribs, restoring some support structure to the lungs. But thoracoplasty was so traumatic, not to say brutal, that it had to be done in two or more stages, prolonging the trauma. Its proponents claimed a "cure" rate varying from 34 to 36.6 percent. But what constitutes a cure is open to varying interpretation: postoperative mortality from thoracoplasty ranged from 10 to 40 percent.

In fact, through all the decades of its ascendancy, surgery remained controversial, a source of nagging uneasiness among doctors. John Alexander, perhaps America's leading thoracic surgeon in the years after World War I, wrote an influential manual, *The Collapse Therapy of Pulmonary Tuberculosis*, which went through a number of editions in the 1930s and in which Alexander staunchly maintained the preeminent value of surgical measures. But others remained dubious. The Trudeau Sanatorium, for instance, adopted pneumothorax, but persistently refrained from performing major operations on its own grounds: candidates for thoracoplasty were sent to Saranac Lake General Hospital. And skeptical evaluations kept appearing in the journals. It was hard to establish a clear connection between collapse therapy and subsequent improvements or relapses. If the patient got better, was that a tribute to the operation or his own resiliency; if he sickened or died, was it the fault of pneumothorax or his own constitution? Satisfactory scientific proof was elusive, since every case was different, and doctors disagreed about what constituted a successful collapse and a favorable outcome; control groups were hard to put together, since nobody could claim patients who didn't undergo surgery were in comparable condition with those who did. A cautious and cautionary 1935 study by Andrew Peters pointed out that in only 38 percent of the cases surveyed had it been possible to produce a satisfactory collapse, and in two thirds of these it had been necessary, thanks to complications, to interrupt treatment prematurely. The only favorable statistic Peters was able to produce, an ambiguous one at best, was that, as of 1935, 70 percent of the patients who had undergone pneumothorax were still alive.

In the forties and fifties, as antibiotics ushered out the era of surgery, critics became more and more vocal, though surgeons fought a vigorous rearguard action. As late as 1953, when drug therapy was firmly established, surgeons were still holding their own in panel discussions, blithely speaking of antibiotics as if they were only preludes to an operation:

DR. JONES: Personally, I think if I were going to evaluate a patient, I'd start him off with PAS and streptomycin and re-evaluate him in four months; then I would decide whether or not this patient was doing well enough on that so that I could proceed with surgery.

But the current of history was against them. As early as 1941 Robert Block and W. B. Tucker, in an exhaustive survey of 2,100 scientific papers on pneumothorax published between 1929 and 1939, calculated that fewer than a twentieth of them assessed results, which were simply assumed to be favorable. And by the late 1950s, pneumothorax had fallen into complete disrepute. "The pneumothorax needle," one surgeon wrote decisively in 1959, "was the most dangerous weapon ever placed in the hands of a physician." Upstaged by streptomycin, PAS, and isoniazid, it vanished, surviving in medical textbooks as an accident rather than a deliberate procedure.

Why, then, the enduring and insistent fashion for a therapy so quickly discredited? Perhaps the tone set by James Benjamin Murphy in 1898 offers a clue: impatient with the failure of medicine to discover a cure, doctors felt the urge to assault the enemy head on. Whatever the results, the surgeon was at least (and with a vengeance) *doing* something. The tubercle bacillus had proved doggedly resistant to assault, and the only alternative left was to work on the victim. And the war, particularly in Europe, may have been a factor. It had produced an alarming upsurge in the new case rate, thanks to disrupted living conditions, and radical solutions seemed necessary; perhaps the extent of its carnage hardened patients and doctors alike to the blood and pain of surgery, which no longer seemed so shocking—to great evils, heroic countermeasures. Whatever the reasons, the surgeon's ascendancy generated its own momentum in the twenties and thirties and fostered a hostility to other approaches. Alexander Fleming first discovered penicillin at St. Mary's Hospital in London in 1928, but nearly a decade was to elapse before its antibiotic properties were thoroughly investigated. His colleague, Sir Ernst Chain, later attributed the delay to the antagonism of Fleming's immediate superior, Sir Almroth Wright, who in Chain's words "had a rigid outlook on science and for whom the concept of chemotherapy was taboo and treated as such throughout his whole scientific career." And, Chain adds, his "attitude was very common among bacteriologists at the time." Somehow, before the late 1930s, the scientific *Zeitgeist* was impacably opposed to the pill and the syringe, and was friendly to the knife.

This was to soon change. For although surgery held the stage in the early decades of the twentieth century, the search for a magic bullet was proceeding, quietly but relentlessly, behind the scenes. Every once in a while a zealot would rush into print, claiming one substance or another as the bane of consumption, and the scientists, patiently and a little wearily, would take it into the laboratory, resigned in advance to the inevitable. Koch's lymph was only the first of a long series. Creosote was a persistent contender; so was calcium, because it was a component in the walls of tubercles, and hence thought an agent useful in sealing off the germs. Mercury and gold found proponents, probably more because of their mythic connections than their chemical properties. Garlic, onions, and radishes were traditional folk remedies for infection (and in fact useful ones; all possess bacteriostatic properties); but around 1915, onions suddenly rushed into the vanguard and were touted by several writers as a sure cure. W. Lintz attempted to test this theory on some hapless tubercular guinea pigs, but encountered an unexpected hitch. "The guinea pigs," he wrote, "absolutely refused to eat onions, preferring to die rather than eat them." Finally Lintz inoculated the animals with mashed-up onions, but the preparation had no effect on their tuberculosis.

Yet, despite the false hopes, even before World War I research was under way that, had it been single-mindedly and continuously pursued, might have conquered tuberculosis thirty or forty years before it finally succumbed. Working in Paris at the Pasteur Institute around 1915, Élie Metchnikoff had devised the original and unorthodox idea that disease-producing microbes might themselves be subject to infection and destruction by other parasites. He had observed, as had many students of tuberculosis, that healthy animals often harbored pathogenic microbes, yet escaped disease. In a running wager with his students at the institute, he took their throat cultures, betting, always successfully, that he would never fail to find a disease-producing organism, often including the tubercle bacillus. Boris D. Sokoloff, one of his most distinguished students, recalls the lecture that always followed this demonstration:

Now why are these germs that we have found in this young man in this latent or passive state, I ask you? . . . Because of our natural resistance? . . . Or our acquired immunity? Surely that is only a partial answer to our question. There must be another factor which retards the dangerously swift development of germs in the human organism; and that cause must in some way be connected with the presence of other harmless, even friendly bacteria, which exercise a destructive and restricting power over our enemies.

From this principle, Metchnikoff argued that there must, somewhere, exist a microbe that could digest or otherwise destroy the tubercle bacillus's armor, the waxy coating that, researchers thought, rendered it impervious to assault. This hunch led him to beehives: where else would one be more likely to find a microorganism partial to wax? And in the end he found what he was looking for, not in a microbe but in the unlikely guise of a moth, *Galleria mellonella,* the bee moth, whose caterpillar doted on honey. In a little-publicized experiment, Metchnikoff introduced tubercle bacilli into the stomach of this caterpillar and found that its digestive juices rapidly devoured the waxy coating and destroyed the bacilli. Elated, he scoured France for *Galleria mellonella* caterpillars, extracted their digestive juices in the quantities necessary for treatment, and tried the preparation on tubercular guinea pigs.

It cured them. But, amazingly, it proved impossible for financial reasons to procure the caterpillars in sufficient quantity to pursue the experiments. World War I, no doubt, diverted both attention and funds from the project; Metchnikoff himself died in 1916 and so was unable to pursue it after Versailles. The gods of fame had not favored him as lavishly as they had Koch. And he was not alone; at roughly the same time other tentative forays into antibiotic research had opened promising channels, which, after an initial freshet, rapidly dried up. As early as 1910, and also at the Pasteur Institute, A. Vandremer had observed that tuberculin lost its activity when added to an extract of *penicillium glaucam.* Isoniazid, the synthesized antibiotic that was, in combination with other drugs, to conquer tuberculosis in the 1950s, first made its appearance in a laboratory in 1912, though its potential was left unexplored. In 1921 a series of experiments at the Pasteur Institute established that a pus-producing microbe, *bacillus pyocaneus,* also released a substance that destroyed cholera and diphtheria bacteria. It was in 1922 that Alexander Fleming first accidentally discovered a germicidal agent in human saliva; almost simultaneously two other researchers, working independently, found two molds, *streptothrix* and *penicillium,* attacking and destroying experimental cultures of *staphylococcus aureus.* Shortly afterward Fleming, once again by accident, observed the same phenomenon, but, strangely, it failed to strike him: "When I saw the bacteria fading away, . . . I had no suspicion that I had a clue to the most powerful therapeutic substance yet found to defeat bacterial infections in the human body."

No theoretical breakthrough, no revolutionary technology needed unearthing for these early discoveries to bear clinical fruit; both the idea behind antibiotic therapy and the laboratory methods necessary to produce it were in place by 1910. Trudeau himself experimented with Koch's lymph in the forlorn hope of finding in it some antibiotic effect and, despite that discouragement died in 1915 believing that ultimately some such substance, effective against consumption, would come to light. But something other than deficient knowledge or lack of technical know-how kept the scientists of the twenties and thirties from pursuing this new trail so tantalizingly opened up; the block must have been ideological or a result of accident rather than the want of a theory. Sokoloff suggests the delay was, oddly, moral: scientists were reluctant, he thinks, to fight disease *with* disease, as if it amounted to counterinsurgency or espionage, abandoning the noble purity of medicine to play tricks on the enemy. Microbes had, after a generation of research, emerged in both the professional and the popular imagination as tiny, sinister gremlins—Marshall McClintock's cure-cottage landlady in Saranac Lake firmly asserted that she had seen the tubercle bacillus under a microscope and that it had claws and a big mouth. Neither the public nor, surprisingly, the elite were prepared to recast the creature so recently identified as the villain in the role of possible savior.

Then, of course, World War I no doubt broke some of the momentum of research. The sanatorium routine and the most common surgical techniques were well established before its outbreak and had only to maintain themselves through the dislocations of the war years, but research into antibiotics had barely begun and hadn't attained the critical mass that would guarantee continuation. Moreover, the one research project sustained through the war collapsed shortly afterward, and this perhaps further discouraged researchers of similar bent. Working in France on a strain of bovine tubercle bacilli, Albert Calmette and his assistant, Camille Guérin, found that, as they recultured the organisms, each successive generation grew less and less virulent. They surmised that they might eventually breed all virulence out of the strain, then use it for vaccinations in the hope of producing immunity. They held to the project throughout the war and by 1919 thought they had bred organisms harmless enough to be used in a live vaccine.

But their research came under quick attack. Some critics questioned their methods; others claimed to have grown virulent strains from samples of the so-called BCG (for "Bacille Calmette-Guérin") culture. Then, in 1930, 249 babies in the North German city of Lübeck were given oral doses of BCG vaccine in the hope of immunizing them. Within months sixty-seven were dead of acute tuberculosis, and the ensuing furor doomed the vaccine, even though an inquiry exonerated it—astonishingly, it turned out that a live culture of virulent tubercle bacilli had been stored in the same incubator with the BCG vaccine and contaminated it. But the storm of publicity following the debacle so poisoned the atmosphere that BCG, despite considerable evidence that it does, at least sometimes, confer immunity against consumption, never recovered its reputation. Even today it provokes controversy among tuberculosis experts and kindles passion, some advocating it for Third World nations still afflicted by major tuberculosis outbreaks, others impugning it. Whatever the merits, the Lübeck disaster clearly embarrassed bacteriological research and may have further discouraged the search for a nonsurgical cure.

It was not until the late thirties that all these embryonic theories were to mature, and broken threads of promising research rejoined. In 1938, with the shadow of another war falling over Europe, the prejudice against antibiotics began to melt away, and Sir Ernst Chain took up Fleming's more-or-less abandoned work, determined to explore the bactericidal possibilities of *penicillium glaucam.* Like Koch's first experiments with the tubercle bacillus, early work went haltingly, primarily because of the temperamental nature of the organisms involved. Staphylococcus, the bacterium against which penicillin first proved effective, grows most profusely at a temperature of about thirty-seven degrees centigrade; but penicillin is liveliest at twenty-four degrees and is only active against bacteria when they are still growing, dividing, and capable of undergoing at least one cell division. Fleming's discovery was pure accident—he had left his staphylococcus cultures out for weeks at a temperature varying between eighteen and twenty degrees, which allowed the *penicillium* to grow but prevented the staphylococcus cultures from developing to maturity, thus keeping them susceptible to the invading mold's bacteriostatic action. It proved tedious and difficult to discover these facts in Chain's laboratory, but when they finally came to light, progress was rapid, and by the early forties the age of miracle drugs had been launched. A massive manufacturing project began, its site shifted to the United States because of the uncertainties of war in Britain. Penicillin flooded the world, and hitherto intractable diseases collapsed: bacterial pneumonia, gonorrhea, syphilis, septicemia.

But not tuberculosis. Early hopes were dashed when penicillin failed to affect it; it became clear that the new drug worked against only the so-called "Gram-positive" bacteria—streptococcus, staphylococcus, pneumococcus. At first researchers thought the tubercle bacillus's waxy coating might be resisting penicillin; later it turned out that Gram-negative bacteria, including the tubercle bacillus, produce an enzyme that destroys penicillin. But the search for an antibiotic capable of overcoming *mycobacterium tuberculosis*'s defenses kept on, now that the principle had been established. And there was reason for hope, since experiments dating back to the years before World War I had repeatedly shown that the tubercle bacillus, in the laboratory at least, was susceptible to the by-products of various fungi and even of other bacteria.

Matters remained there, however, until 1943, when a New Jersey chicken farmer, puzzled and upset by an infection that his birds seemed to be acquiring from the dirt in their barnyard, brought them to Selman Waksman's laboratory at Rutgers University. The confrontation seems an unlikely one, the distressed poultryman and the Ukrainian-born cosmopolitan microbiologist, but it proved productive. Waksman and his coworkers soon established that the offending microorganism was a mold of the genus *streptomyces;* experiments showed that, like *penicillium,* it generated antibacterial by-products, with the exciting difference that it was strikingly effective against Gram-negative bacteria, including the tubercle bacillus. The fiftieth anniversary of Koch's lymph had just passed, so all the participants were acutely sensitive to the need for caution as well as speed, but research progressed rapidly in spite of the difficulty of producing the new drug in adequate quantities for experiment. By 1944 enough of it was available to conduct a test on twenty tubercular guinea pigs, and the results were startling: all ten of the animals given the drug improved, with traces of illness absent or barely detectable after a few weeks.

By 1946 human experiments were well under way. Sixteen patients with pulmonary tuberculosis at the Mayo Clinic had taken streptomycin and shown marked improvement; large and growing lung lesions had promptly improved and occasionally healed. Scenting a bonanza, six drug companies (Abbott, Lilly, Merck, Pfizer, Squibb, and Upjohn) sponsored a nationwide study, donating a large quantity of the new drug to the American Trudeau Society (the medical wing of the National Tuberculosis Association) for experimental use at sanatoriums. Various doses were tested, results in patients measured, effects on cultures of tubercle bacilli assessed. At the Olive View Sanatorium in California, 110 patients received streptomycin, while 100 more were left as controls (either because they were taking other experimental drugs or, as the report ominously put it, because "they were deliberately set aside as controls"). The lucky recipients improved sharply. They coughed and spit less, their fevers fell, the bacteria counts in their sputum samples declined, and, gradually, their X rays improved. But their spirits soared, with a vigor "quite disproportionate to the meager effect shown on serial roentgenograms": somehow the expectation of miracles was thick in the air, slow though they were in coming. At the Trudeau Sanatorium, of thirty-five patients given streptomycin, twenty-seven improved within the course of a year, beginning in December 1946 and ending in November 1947.

Excitement and publicity mounted, but to nothing like the pitch of hysteria Robert Koch had provoked in 1890. For in the intervening years the crusade against consumption had institutionalized itself, replacing the *grandes gestes* of self-appointed heroes with a perhaps duller but certainly safer ethic of gradual, collective effort. Even the earliest research on streptomycin was shared, Waksman dividing the credit with his colleagues, Elizabeth Bugie and Albert Schatz, and by the time the drug went into clinical trials, responsibility had dispersed among virtually all the leading medical figures in the antituberculosis crusade. Tests were conducted everywhere, following every imaginable scheme, and the air of caution was perhaps the easier to maintain because the tide of news, good and bad, was not surging around any single figure, as had been the case with Koch and Calmette. This proved the wiser in that, as work proceeded, streptomycin's undesirable side effects surfaced. It could cause mild malaise and muscle aches; some patients resuming therapy after a few weeks' lapse experienced violent febrile reactions. And streptomycin could also attack the inner and middle ear, causing temporary deafness and vertigo.

But the worst drawback was one destined to plague antibiotics through the rest of their history—resistance. Despite the enthusiasm of the earliest field reports, streptomycin, though it sometimes relieved symptoms with dramatic quickness, worked only slowly against the tubercle bacillus, whose sluggish metabolism proved its strongest defense. The drug operated almost passively, interfering with the growth and reproduction of the tubercle bacillus rather than attacking it outright; it was largely ineffective during the considerable periods when the organism was dormant, and this meant that for effective treatment the dosage had to be continued for months. That in turn allowed resistant strains of bacteria to develop. At the Trudeau Sanatorium an early study concluded that resistance began to appear during the fourth week of treatment and increased steadily thereafter. The early upsurge of hope, without ever entirely receding, had by 1948 come to include a new kind of despair, and it invented, in the midst of the optimism, a new kind of agony for the patient schooled from the story of penicillin to expect dramatic final victories. Instead, like Paul Davenant, the postwar lunger in A. E. Ellis's novel *The Rack,* the patient faced a new sophisticated form of the old mouse-against-cat battle with the disease, an initial surge of improvement, then a sudden dispiriting stagnation, followed by the suspenseful wait, since it took some time for the cultures to be tested by which he could tell if he'd developed resistance. Such failure of the drug inevitably meant a return to the racking inventory of earlier surgical procedures—pneumothorax, lung resection, thoracoplasty.

But by 1949 a new antibiotic, PAS (para-aminosalicylic acid), which had first been used in Sweden in 1943 and had been widely tested after 1945, proved its effectiveness. Doctors quickly recognized that, if combined with streptomycin, it could inhibit the strains of bacteria that developed resistance to streptomycin, and vice versa. A new era of combination therapy, even today essential in the treatment of tuberculosis, had been born. The enemy was destined never to be conquered with a single devastating weapon but always held at bay by a variety of partly successful therapies. PAS stepped in where streptomycin failed; the damage drugs didn't repair could be remedied surgically; whatever debilitation remained could be fought by the old but still psychologically potent forces of rest, good food, a heartening view, pure air, and optimism. At the annual meetings of the Trudeau Society, even as late as the close of the 1940s and the early 1950s, no one envisioned the disappearance of surgery or the ultimate closing of the sanatoriums: the enemy had been fought to a truce but not beyond. In 1952 the society, with at least seeming confidence, issued an official statement endorsing rest: "There has been no clear indication that in advanced cases of tuberculosis the amount of rest therapy"—and that, of course, included the various forms of lung-immobilizing surgery as well as bed rest—"may be reduced with impunity even with fairly effective drug treatment." Oddly, Mrs. Shannon in Saranac Lake, disturbed at the empty beds in her rest cottage and writing in anguish to the governor that same year, was more in touch with the realities, or at least more willing to face them, than the leaders of the crusade.

And, though she could not have known it, the final, decisive blow was about to be struck. On January 19, 1952, two rival sets of papers arrived at the offices of the *American Review of Tuberculosis,* originating from two keenly competing drug companies, Squibb and Hoffmann–La Roche; their simultaneity attested to the fierceness of the race and the importance of the stakes. The papers, printed in the *Review*'s April 1952 issue, announced a new antituberculosis drug, isonicotinic acid hydrazide. Hoffmann–La Roche dubbed it Rimifon; Squibb called it Nydrazid; generic names eventually to dominate were isoniazid, IAH, and INH. But the reports, describing the compound and a closely related one, called Marsilid by Hoffmann–La Roche and Iproniazid by Squibb, promised spectacular results. Edward H. Robitzek and Irving V. Selikoff, two Squibb researchers, announced that they had given the new drugs to ninety-seven patients at the Sea View Sanatorium on Staten Island, with results so astonishing that they were barely able to maintain the sober prose demanded in a scientific journal; their enthusiasm shone discreetly but unmistakably through the deceptively deadpan tone of their case histories:

CASE 3 (K.R.). This 24-year-old Negro female was admitted to Sea View Hospital on November 7, 1951. Although symptoms of her pulmonary tuberculosis were first noted in 1948, there was marked exacerbation in October 1951. On admission to Sea View Hospital on November 7, 1951, her status was critical. In the previous months her weight had decreased from a normal of 125 pounds to approximately 80 pounds. She was highly toxic and had been amenorrheic since early 1951. Marked anorexia, lethargy, and weakness, and [a] moderately severe cough and expectoration were present. Her temperatures ranged from 103° to 104°F. There was persistent diarrhea, possibly due to tuberculous enteritis. . . . The sputum was highly positive for acid-fast bacilli on every examination.

Therapy with . . . Marsilid was begun on November 24, 1951, at 4 mg. per kg. per day. Within a few days, the patient's temperature began to descend and reached normal in ten days. At the same time there was a complete reversal in this patient's clinical state. Her appetite became ravenous. Diarrhea subsided completely within two weeks. The edema disappeared promptly during the first week of therapy. There was a remarkable gain in well-being. Four weeks after the onset of therapy, cough and expectoration had almost completely disappeared. Rapid weight gain was noted and after eight weeks of therapy approximately a 37-pound gain in weight was noted. . . .

Two sputum examinations in the first two weeks of therapy were positive for acid-fast bacilli. However, the following week, [the] smear of the sputum was negative for tubercle bacilli and five subsequent consecutive examinations have been negative. . . . A roentgenogram on January 7, 1952 showed marked improvement. . . . The multiple cavities present in the left lung were all much smaller. The patient is continuing to receive therapy and is clini-

cally completely asymptomatic, without cough or expectoration and with excellent appetite. She feels strong and
is at normal weight.

Needless to say, the popular press soon scented such reports
out, the more easily in that the tests had been conducted not
at Saranac or in any of the other relatively remote centers but
on Staten Island. Newspaper photos appeared showing Marsilid patients, not long since supine, hopeless, and anorexic,
now dancing in the aisles of their sanatoriums.

The bulk of professional opinion was, with reason, more
conservative. It was quickly realized that the ebullience of
patients taking Marsilid (or iproniazid, as it came to be called
generically) was not solely the result of its bacteriostatic properties. It turned out to be a powerful stimulant, capable in
some instances of causing psychotic behavior. Though patients
felt immediately better when they took it, developed insatia-
ble appetites, and gained weight posthaste, they also experienced withdrawal symptoms when they were taken off it,
as a Yale study at New Haven's Laurel Heights Sanatorium
established. The drug quickly disappeared from the market,
replaced permanently by isoniazid; while its results were not
so immediately spectacular, it emerged over the course of the
next year that it was, when used in combination with streptomycin or PAS, the most effective of all the antitubercular
drugs. Used together with streptomycin, a 1953 study concluded, it had not merely bacteriostatic effects, inhibiting the
germs, but bactericidal ones, killing them outright. Squibb
began advertising it as more potent against the tubercle bacillus than any other known compound, better able as it was to
penetrate the barriers posed by the necrotic tissue of tubercles, and by the cell walls of the phagocytes within which
tubercle bacilli are able to survive.

The story of how this suddenly rediscovered drug, known
since 1912, came to be recognized as antitubercular is an interesting one, a story of indirection, told by H. Herbert Fox, a
Hoffmann–La Roche scientist, in the August 8, 1952, issue of

Science. As early as 1945, researchers had discovered that one of the B vitamins, nicotinamide, was slightly active against tuberculosis. It was not by itself powerful enough to compete with streptomycin against the disease, but it suggested the intriguing possibility that vitamins might work in some hitherto unknown way against the tubercle bacillus. Research quickly proved it wasn't the vitamin activity of the compound that fought the microbes, but something else, and biochemists and pharmacologists successfully began putting in some molecules and pulling others out in the hope of locating and perhaps intensifying the germicidal component.

Scientific caution counterbalanced the clamor of the mass media, and for the next year or so the studies of isoniazid, alone and in combination with PAS and streptomycin, took care to preserve not merely the appearance of understatement but the reality of it; they carefully suppressed the excitement the authors of the Sea View study had, no doubt inadvertently, let show. But it nonetheless was dawning on the leaders of the antituberculosis crusade that, in America at least, the end was at hand; the era of the sanatorium and the TB surgeon were both drawing to an end. One by one, the patients left their sanatoriums; the surgical scars healed, not to be replaced by new ones. Once more Isabel Smith, Trudeau's model patient in 1937, appeared in the pages of *Life* magazine, but in a new context—an article announcing the closing of the Trudeau: "A Victim of Progress: Sanatorium Closes on Optimistic Note." She had left the hospital, married, moved to an apartment in Saranac Lake, and by the fall of 1954 was busy writing her life story, *Wish I Might. Life* caught the few remaining patients and staff as they rattled disconsolately about the hospital in its last few days. A nurse, Marie Miller, gazed at a row of empty clipboards for patient records on the infirmary wall. Alma Pierce, the occupational therapy teacher, sat in her deserted workshop: "I guess I'll go home to Brooklyn." Irene Bloomer, a patient, waited for her husband to take her to Ray Brook Sanatorium, the state hospital down the road. Larry Doyle, once a New York Giants second baseman and a Trudeau inmate since 1942, ate his last meal at the head of an otherwise empty table. They left, the gates closed behind them, and *Life* gave its readers a last elegiac glance at the statue of the founder.

> Only the recumbent figure of Edward Trudeau remained,
> . . . resting beneath his blanket of bronze on which winter
> now had spread a softer shroud.

One by one, in and around Saranac and throughout the nation, the other sanatoriums and cure cottages gradually followed Trudeau's lead: it was a pioneer at the end of the crusade as it had been at the beginning. Some small private and some large state institutions hung on. A few elderly patients were too infirm, physically or mentally, ever to adjust to life on the outside: the sanatorium had become their world, and existence was unimaginable elsewhere. In 1961 the Sanatorium Gabriels, a small religious institution outside Saranac Lake run by the Sisters of Mercy, was still open, caring for eight patients, all between the ages of seventy-one and eighty-one. The last New York state sanatorium, Homer Folks in Oneonta, closed in 1973.

But for all practical purposes, by 1960 the American sanatorium had vanished from the landscape. Some, like the Loomis Sanatorium in the Catskills, fell into the hands of private entrepreneurs; others, like Mount McGregor and Ray Brook, made ideal prisons; more came to lead a natural and comparatively dignified existence as residential health care facilities or nursing homes—Gaylord Farm, in fact, still functions as a rehabilitation center. Saranac Lake remembers the White Plague; that, after all, was its history. But the rest of the country made haste to forget. Tuberculosis still kills four of every 100,000 Americans; it is still a major threat to the ill housed and ill fed; recently it has gained a new foothold as one of the opportunistic infections attacking AIDS patients. And worldwide four million people catch it each year, and a million die of it. But it has disappeared from American consciousness, and American conscience. "The cluster of metaphors and attitudes formerly attached to TB," Susan Sontag recently wrote, "split up and are parceled out to two diseases": insanity and cancer.

Yet acts of amnesia are rarely so complete. Sleeping porches—now used as studies, sewing rooms, or repositories for junk—still quietly recall the era of the crusade in hundreds of thousands of American homes built between the first and second world wars. Antituberculosis health routines, like sleeping with an open window, were an integral part of school health curriculums well into the 1950s. And the National Tuberculosis Association has survived as the American Lung Association.

Yet long after they were closed, the hospitals themselves could send a primal chill even through those happily ignorant of the disease they were built to fight. In Kansas City, Missouri, in the mid-1960s, a ritual of adolescence was a visit to the "Haunted Hospital," the abandoned Kansas City tuberculosis sanatorium southeast of the city, on the road to Independence. It stood in remote country, atop a wooded hill, at the end of a long road that ended at a chain link fence threateningly studded with "NO TRESPASSING" signs. The windows on the sleeping porches were broken and gaping; the building had become a way station for derelicts. Most adolescents prudently carried their rebellion only as far as the gate, cowed by parental warnings against an unnamed, dreaded, inevitably fatal disease. When you went to the hospital as a patient, they recalled, you never came out. The illness was a death sentence, and it echoed loudly even among a generation that had forgotten its name and had no direct knowledge of its terrors. The braver souls who actually broke into the hospital building came back with tales of a door blazoned "MORGUE," of drains in the floors, immediately identified as conduits for gushing blood. And everywhere, though invisible, were the germs, long idle but still potent, waiting to leap up and seize the foolhardy intruder. So when you went home, after the exhilarating terrors of the visit itself, you had weeks of a subtler but longer-lived panic, awaiting the appearance of symptoms whose nature you couldn't anticipate. Any new sensation you felt, any small bodily change, might, of course, be only an earnest of your progressing adolescence, your advancing sexual maturity. But it might also be a herald of doom, death, the blasting of hopes, the end of everything, and this possibility was at least as titillating as it was fearsome.

In a generation ignorant of its symptoms, even of its name, consumption ironically survived, not as a physical threat but as a symbol, perhaps the more powerful because it bore no label. The War on Consumption had spent three generations demythologizing the disease, doggedly routing miasmic vapors with onslaughts of fact. But no sooner had the enemy been defeated than the myths, if in attenuated form, fluttered back in, and mid-American teenagers in the 1960s found themselves (though it's unlikely they knew it) psychically at one with Henri Murger's Francine, doomed and eroticized by her consumption:

> "You will last till to-morrow," said the Doctor. "You have one more night left to live."
> "Thank Heaven," said the girl, "it's winter, and the nights are long."

For most of its visitors, of course, the Haunted Hospital breathed only a hint of these potent myths; most never dared take the plunge into its depth. Two veterans of one such mid-sixties foray into the grounds made it only to the warning-studded gate at the top of the hill. They looked at the mustard-colored stucco of the main building; at the gaping broken windows; they thought about the germs that, according to their parents, had been there for years and would remain there for years.

Then one of them looked up and saw, hanging low on the branch of a tree on the grounds, a coat, whipping and clawing in the wind.

With one accord, they leapt into their car and sped home.

10

Illness Imagined

In 1665, a plague year, the Black Death swept across the Continent and through Britain in what was to be one of its last major visitations. It arrived in London that April, and mortality from it peaked in September. Panic spread; the city emptied, and everyone who could afford to bolted for the countryside. Pepys, confined to London by his duties as a rising civil servant, recorded some of the horrors in a breathless, headlong diary entry:

> My meeting dead corpses of the plague, carried to be buried close to me at noonday through the City in Fenchurch Street. To see a person sick of the sores carried close by me by Grace Church in a hackney-coach. My finding the Angel Tavern at the lower end of Tower Hill shut up; and more than that, the alehouse at Tower Stairs; and more than that, that the person was then dying of the plague when I was last there, . . . and I overheard the mistress of the house saying sadly to her husband somebody was very ill, but did not think it was of the plague. To hear that poor Payne my waterman hath buried a child and is dying himself. To hear that a laborer I sent but the

other day to Dagenhams to know how they did there is dead of the plague; and that one of my own watermen, that carried me daily, fell sick as soon as he had landed me Friday morning last, when I had been all night upon the water (and I believed he did get his infection that day at Brainford) is now dead of the plague. . . . To hear that Mr. Lewes hath another daughter sick. And lastly, that both my servants, W. Hewers and Tom Edwards, have lost their fathers . . . this week—doth put me into great apprehensions of melancholy, and with good reason.

Each week London printed a Bill of Mortality; a selection from the one issued the week of September 12, 1665, shows some of the larger picture, the dark reality against which Pepys's personal griefs and fears stood out. The list was alphabetical, by disease.

Aged	43
Burnt in his Bed by a Candle at St. Giles Cripplegate	1
Consumption	134
Feaver	309
Grief	3
Griping in the Guts	51
Plague	7165
Spotted Feaver	101
Surfeit	49
Wormes	15

At the distance of three centuries, the mingling here of ruthless fact with apparent fantasy is disconcerting. It was the beginning of the age of science, an era of rational investigation of which, indeed, Pepys himself was an enthusiastic proponent—he had been elected as a Fellow of the Royal Society in February of that year. And some of the entries in the bill no modern epidemiologist would dispute. The symptoms of plague are unmistakable; we can, even at our remove, accept the tally of 7,165 deaths that week as implicitly reliable, safely empirical. But who, in the twentieth century, dies of grief? Of surfeit? And if these on the one hand seem too imaginative, too fanciful, even too romantic for clinical discourse, "Griping in the Guts" seems too earthy, too immediate; "Feaver" too vague; "Consumption," granted how little was known in 1665 of its pathology, much less its cause, an unreliable diagnosis at best. On the one hand Pepys reaches compulsively after specifics—the corpses carried through the streets to burial at broad noon, the very place where the stricken waterman caught the disease. Why, then, with his nervous, omnivorous eye didn't he or anyone else of decisive influence notice the rats and the fleas? The seventeenth-century mind was at once more specific (who would now reserve a separate entry for the man "Burnt in his Bed by a Candle at St. Giles Cripplegate"?) and less specific (what *kinds* of "Wormes"?) than our own; where we see nothing, it ran riot; where facts shout at us, it went stone deaf.

This is only a glimpse, yet it reveals how definitive the imagination can be, even in realms that present themselves at first as domains of hard, empirical fact. There is no apparent reason why Pepys, his contemporaries, or for that matter his forebears might not have turned their attention to the vermin swarming off ships newly arrived from plague-stricken ports. Even in the Middle Ages, authorities responsible for public health had realized that the illness was spreading on shipboard from infected localities to clear ones; the quarantines they established show how close they were to recognizing the real source of the disease. Leeuwenhoek's famous letter to the Royal Society describing the microorganisms he'd seen through the microscope postdated this last great sweep of the plague by only eleven years; no insurmountable impediment to his discovery existed fifty years before. It was simply that the European imagination, collective and individual, was unwilling, unready, to think epidemiologically or bacteriologically. It was otherwise disposed; the kind of statistical thinking that would allow accurate studies of the spread of contagion lay in the future. Because they saw illness differently, it was different.

At this remove, and clothed as our imaginations now are in the regalia of science, such thinking seems at best naïve, at

275

worst perverse, and the course of history that led away from it appears inevitable, the fated triumph of fact over myth. We can thus cast a critical eye on the Bills of Mortality, relatively sure, for example, that many of the 134 deaths attributed to "Consumption" were otherwise caused; just as sure that some of those set down to "Grief" or "Surfeit" were in fact tuberculosis. It feels like relief to cast off the shackles of myth and wander free in the light of Truth. Small wonder that in her recent and influential essay, *Illness as Metaphor,* Susan Sontag bridled at the human propensity to encrust facts with encumbering layers of metaphor. It seems, she argues, particularly unfair to the person struck by illness, who, already burdened by the sufferings of the disease, has to shoulder as well the added load of collective hallucinations about it:

> Trying to comprehend "radical" or "absolute" evil, we search for adequate metaphors. But the modern disease metaphors are all cheap shots. The people who have the real disease are also hardly helped by hearing their disease's name constantly being dropped as the epitome of evil.

But does the modern understanding of illness really rest on a bedrock of fact? Consider the case of tuberculosis, the disease now so thoroughly mastered by science that, according to Sontag, cancer had to be summoned up to replace it as an overdetermined, metaphor-laden plague. The triumph medical science won over it is unmistakable, and yet think how much mystery this two-centuries-long march of enlightenment left unsolved. In America the disease has been nearly forgotten, so absolute was the victory against it, yet it would be no exaggeration to say that what we don't know about it even now outscales what we do. We don't know for sure why (or even that) the long epidemic wave of tuberculosis apparently now ending began in the late seventeenth century. We don't know why certain strains of the tubercle bacillus cause disease while other strains remain perfectly harmless; nor are the biochemical or behavioral differences between the two fully understood. It has never been entirely settled how tuberculosis is most often transmitted, whether on droplets of liquid or particles of dry dust. It isn't known why, once infected, some people come down with clinical tuberculosis while others fight the disease off and remain healthy. No one knows for sure why the apices of the lungs are the most frequent sites of infection among those in whom the disease reaches an acute state—it used to be thought this area was vulnerable because of its high concentration of oxygen, but that has been disputed. Once tubercles appear, we don't know why some of them are caseous (or cheesy) in consistency, while others calcify.

No wonder that debate smoldered for decades over exactly what constituted a reliable diagnosis of active pulmonary tuberculosis. Nineteenth-century physicians relied on the often ambiguous and impenetrable sounds they heard in their patients' chests, but even the advent of new diagnostic tools failed to settle the problem. A positive Mantoux test meant only that one had been exposed, and X rays were—and are—subject to disagreeing interpretations. When they were first introduced in 1896, by Dr. Francis H. Williams of Boston, a respondent to his paper expressed a widely shared medical sentiment:

> Frank Williams has just shown you some plates and tells you that the heart is here and the lung is here. Now I can't see a thing in these plates, and to be truthful I don't think that he can.

Nor did doubt end with diagnosis. The whole enormous economy of the antituberculosis movement rose, flourished, and vanished without ever clearly establishing its efficacy against the disease. It's never been proved whether or not the rest cure worked. Pneumothorax, widespread though it was by the 1930s and confident though its advocates were, remained controversial, and it was never scientifically established that the procedure in fact retarded the spread of the disease. Still less did the more heroic operations like thoracoplasty ever

prove their value; though their formidably skilled practitioners would no doubt have been horrified to know it, they were
destined to disappear as completely from the medical armory
as onion juice and arsenic. Authorities on the subject have
never fully agreed whether or not BCG vaccine produces immunity against tuberculosis, a subject that still arouses pas-
sions, since an effective vaccine would be the best weapon
against tuberculosis in Third World countries, where the elaborate and long-drawn-out antibiotic regimen is difficult to implement.

Even the effective antituberculosis drugs, streptomycin,
PAS, isoniazid, and a later generation of still-more-effective
compounds (rifampin is the most important of these) work
their magic at least partly in secret. When the earliest antibiotics like penicillin failed to affect the microbes, experimenters theorized that its waxy coating protected the bacillus
against it, and that hence only a fat-soluble substance, able to
penetrate its armor, would work. Yet the drugs that finally
won the victory were, against the predictions, water soluble.
Opinion varied for years about how far the successful drugs
operated in killing the bacterium and how far they merely
inhibited its growth and reproduction. Even today opinion
varies about the optimum combination of drugs, the optimum dosage, the optimum period over which the treatment
should be continued.

Consumption, in short, yielded its hegemony without giving
up its mystery, and the triumph of the antituberculosis crusade
was more complete in its results than it was in exposing the
enemy's secrets. The movement coasted from success to success along a course of aptly chosen metaphors, on images of
sickness and health created by its leaders. As far as possible, of
course, these images followed, or at least didn't blatantly con-
tradict, hard-won empirical knowledge. But neither were they
enslaved to it; they were as much the product of vision as
research and were invented not solely by scientists, nor yet by
philanthropists and publicists; the tubercular contributed as
well. Though the story doesn't lack for individual heroes—

Koch, Trudeau, Knopf, perhaps even Biggs—it is largely a collective one, and it was in this direction the historical momentum lay. The Health Heroes, as Metropolitan Life dubbed them in its pamphlet series, were early pioneers; the decisive later advances were all group efforts. Koch's name was and to some extent still is a household word, but what about Selman Waksman, who surely contributed as much or more to the victory? The sanatorium, planned community that it was, framed the cure as a group effort, and the metaphors invoked for it, whether by doctors, planners, or patients, were all communal: the town, the school, the family.

If, so far in this century, the dominant trend in the medical profession has been toward specialization and centralization, each mode of treatment restricted to the smallest and most carefully controlled group possible, the War on Consumption was a detour in another direction. Though they were sorely tempted, at the founding of the national association in 1904, to oust laymen from control of the movement, the physicians relented, and at least until the antibiotics remedicalized the battle against tuberculosis, it was an effort in which science participated but didn't dominate. A conventional view of modern medical history draws a contrast between the old-fashioned doctor, steeped in intuition, a natural comforter and master of the bedside manner, and the coldhearted technocrat, measuring symptoms and interpreting test results. But in Saranac Lake (to cite the paradigm) a third pattern emerged, perhaps best exemplified in Lawrason Brown. To his patients and the townspeople, he was a reassuringly folksy figure, shuffling through the streets in his bedroom slippers, dispensing medicine, warnings, charity, and solace where each was appropriate. Yet, Norman Rockwell small-town doctor though he may have appeared, he was one of the leaders of his profession, a scholarly and even compulsive researcher, who served as president of the National Tuberculosis Association in 1923 and 1924 and who did more to codify and systematize the rest cure than any other figure. Nor was this an extraordinary catholicity of ability on his part; it was simply that the movement, blending science and art, specialization and nonspecialization, did not force on him the choices more typical of his profession in the later twentieth century.

By tacit collective assent, the leaders of the crusade made its battles everyman's, as indeed the instigators of the first crusades had. As soon as it became known that the disease was spread by a microbe, the temptation arose to quarantine the victims, sequestering them from the general population as completely and irrevocably as lepers had been in the Middle Ages. But instead the whole nation chose to shoulder the burden of the disease, taking precautions against its spread, but not isolating its victims completely. The modus vivendi between the sick and the well at Saranac was simply a paradigm of the way the nation as a whole learned to live with tuberculosis. To get it was a special fate, and to treat it became a specialty; but neither the fate nor the medical response to it were allowed to sunder themselves entirely from the communal life of the nation. Sanatoriums were not hospitals; their routines were the distilled essence of normal life, not a clinical regimen disruptively substituted for it. In that sense the metaphors of battle and struggle most often chosen by the antituberculosis effort were deceptive. For much of the battle lay, in the preantibiotic era, in learning how to live with the disease, to accept it as woven in with the rest of life, and to outgrow the natural desire to view it as an untoward bolt of nemesis.

Edward Livingston Trudeau insisted explicitly on this in *An Autobiography*:

> I have had ample opportunity in the past forty years to get used to illness and suffering; but it took me a long time to learn, imperfectly though it be, that acquiescence is the only way for the tuberculous invalid to conquer fate. To cease to rebel and struggle, and to learn to be content with part of a loaf when one cannot have a whole loaf, though a hard lesson to learn, is good philosophy for the tuberculous invalid, and to his astonishment he often finds that what he considers the half-loaf, when acquiesced in, proves most satisfying.

The very inconsistency of this statement is therapeutic: a battle whose most potent martial weapon is acquiescence. By fictionalizing tuberculosis in this way, Trudeau and his followers were finding a way to link the enforced idleness of the disease to the prevailing American ethos of activity and conquest, clearing a space for the ill amidst a national passion for health. If you drive along the streets of any American city or town, it's hard to mistake the hospital for any other sort of building. It stands out, visibly separate from the rest of the life flowing around it; its functions have been specialized, sequestered, nearly as alien to the normal as secret temple rites. But sanatorium culture avoided sealing itself in therapeutic purdah. Sanatorium architecture, at its best, softened the institutional into the domestic, implementing the former but not breaking with the latter. Logic may find it hard to reconcile such apparent contradictions, but metaphor making finds it easy. Science was ultimately able to vanquish much of the sufferings individuals underwent from this disease, but in the meantime a shared act of imagination allowed them to live with it.

This could, of course, seem intimidating and burdensome, in precisely the ways Susan Sontag describes. A new patient, already debilitated, wrenched rudely away from the familiar and suddenly stripped of his expectations, found himself forced to lead a new and alien way of life. Rules had to be learned and followed. The doctor, hard enough to cope with as a dispenser of medicines, acquired the added intellectual authority of the professor, and the father's familial right to extort emotional blackmail. The landscape, though beautiful, was silent and empty, and from the confines of the hospital bed appeared distant and untouchable. But once they'd passed the initial period of rebellion and readjustment, most patients came to appreciate such initiation rites. The sanatorium didn't allow them to vegetate, passively undergoing the ministrations of the staff; they had to *live,* in circumstances adjusted to the illness, but nonetheless still in touch with normal life.

The postmodern temptation is to read this situation, following Michel Foucault, as an economy of power, both patients and doctors locked in a grid of manipulation of which neither is master, a mere display of symbols and signs whose ultimate end is to dramatize the power of signs *as* signs, rather than the power of what they represent. The subtext, however, of much of Foucault's writing, is an unstated rebellion against such dramas, a suggestion that we'd do well to abandon such semiotic charades, and free ourselves from the dense net of controls in which they entrap us. Such, certainly, is the tenor of his argument in *The Birth of the Clinic* and *Discipline and Punish,* the two books that directly and indirectly explore the relationship between healer and patient. Like Sontag he seems, though less explicitly and more analytically, to be asking us to wrestle ourselves free of the power of the image (though, unlike Sontag, Foucault appears doubtful that there's anything so simple as fact to counterpose against it).

Yet the testimony of sanatorium alumni suggests a less puritanical reading. Even the naïve patients often saw keenly through the artificialness of antitubercular optimism and knew they were participating, half willingly and half reluctantly, in the creation of a fiction. And that awareness held them free of subjugation even as they accepted the benefits. Remember the debate about this subject in the *Journal of the Outdoor Life,* and the surprising awareness of its participants. *As for making believe, why, we start practicing that when we are mere children. . . . If it does the work, doesn't the end for which we are striving, justify the means?* Images need not be imposed one-sidedly on the vulnerable by the powerful; they are not, necessarily, strong stories by the influential that drown out the weaker narratives of the humble. They can also be shared, the products of unspoken negotiation and agreement.

That does not mean the participants always wholly agree or that they are guided by a conscious appreciation of what's best for the commonweal. The story of the crusade is, after all, full of individuals of cranky vision, who, if they had had their way, would have driven the effort in directions amenable to their own demons. Hermann Biggs, much though he contributed to civic antituberculosis programs, would, left to his own devices, have established something like a police state, a Platonic republic ruled by a physician-king. S. Adolphus Knopf, less ambitiously but just as tendentiously, would have had the nation—tubercular and nontubercular alike—plunging daily into a matutinal freezing bath. Bernarr MacFadden would have enforced mile-long runs and a vegetarian diet. But all the ragged ends—scientific, sociological, elitist, and popular—blended over several generations into an imaginative consensus about how we were to live with consumption. No quick cure emerged, so the disease had to be endured. The victims, being contagious, had to be isolated, but not absolutely; they were to remain connected to the body politic. Tuberculosis, once known, quickly emerged as a health crisis of immense proportions. Only half consciously, and as a group, Americans decided to fight against it, but also to accept it. This was no insult to the sick, despite its occasional tyrannies, but an act of wisdom and compassion.

Consider the contrasting case of AIDS, for which, unpredictable as its future may now be, the War on Consumption offers some useful examples. AIDS first appeared in a world permeated by far higher expectations for medicine than were current when Trudeau fell ill in 1872. It had gotten used to immediate and surefire remedies; if a disease appeared, the technological weapons were deployed, and a diagnosis, a prophylaxis, and a cure appeared forthwith. Medicine was held in awe for its proficiency, but the respect it called up, though deep, was narrow, the acclaim due an engineer's finely tuned virtuosity rather than an artist's instinctive feel for the whole of experience. When, for years at a stretch, scientists failed to define the disease satisfactorily and proved unable even to identify a cause organism (as of this writing Koch's Postulates have still not been satisfied for the suspect organism, HIV), much less produce a cure, the failure produced a mounting outrage among much of the gay community. It seemed a further act of rejection against an already marginalized group: how was it that the scientific miracles so readily marshaled against the other great plagues could not be arrayed against this? To gay men the delay in a remedy often seemed an act of discrimination against them; in the public at large, it engendered a fear of the disease's victims, and this served still further to isolate the ill and the groups to which they belonged. The network of social cooperation and tolerance that developed around tuberculosis in the absence of a cure had disappeared; there was no way to think about disease except as a scientific problem, and when science, even temporarily, failed, there was no bulwark against panic and recrimination.

To which, by mid-1987, the nation's media had given full vent. Responsible journals, fortresses of restraint, shuddered at the economic consequences of AIDS, hinted at the need for quarantine, prodded the unquestionable drama of getting and living with the disease into hysterical melodrama. "Plague" rapidly emerged as a favorite term, and writers apparently meant to invoke its apocalyptic connotations as the name for inevitable, universal doom. It is as if, nationally, we had no memory. Much of the panic had been precipitated by a projection that there might be a total of a quarter milion AIDS cases by 1990. And yet a mere fifty years ago, in 1937 alone, toward the end of the epidemic, 112,000 people contracted tuberculosis and nearly 70,000 died of it, among a population barely half the size of the present one. Unlike AIDS, consumption can be contracted casually, by a sneeze; from a loud-voiced preacher, if you sit in the front pew. America once knew, apparently, that what had to be lived with, could be; where we shriek, our parents quietly coped. And the ill were served, not shunned.

From a scientific point of view, the evidence is not indisputable that the rest cure worked against tuberculosis, that the surgery devised for it succeeded in its aim, or even that the segregation of the ill and lessened crowding in the city was the decisive factor in reducing the spread of infection. But the publicity, the widely circulated reassurance that something was being done, that the enemy could be conquered, relieved anxiety for the unaffected and, perhaps more important, made it easier for the stricken to bear their affliction.

In Europe, when Franz Kafka came down with the disease, he was struck by the reticence with which his doctors treated it. "Verbally I don't learn anything definite," he wrote, "since in discussing tuberculosis . . . everybody drops into a shy, evasive, glassy-eyed manner of speech." That was in 1924, and in Europe, where literature had rushed to give consumption an imaginative shape but where in life it apparently remained taboo, forbidden direct access to daily discourse. How different the case was in America, at least in the sanatorium, where there was an arsenal full of ways to think, talk, and even act about it. If you thumbed through your monthly issue of the *Journal of the Outdoor Life,* you could read fellow patients' accounts of their struggles with the "bug," their lives at the "san"; you could read explicit and detailed, though popularly worded, medical lectures by physicians. There were thumbnail biographies of Heroes of Tuberculosis, like Thoreau; note how much more robust a figure he was for the anticonsumption movement than the gossamer invalid who lay on his deathbed in Concord, inspiring Emerson:

> It was fortunate for himself as well as for us that Thoreau cared so much for the outdoor air. In our day we know that a man who has lived out of doors most of his life yet dies of tuberculosis at the age of forty-five, has probably added ten or fifteen years at least to his life. Had he been carried off at thirty, as might not unlikely have been the case if he consented to work indoors, our American literature would have been without one of its deepest well springs of originality.

Yet, of course, such profusion, such explicitness, had its drawbacks. The strength of scientific medicine is that it brings to a specific problem a specific cure, clean and definite. Its weakness, correspondingly, is that when it fails it leaves us with nothing to hold onto, no residue of mystical hope. Metaphor and imagination, on the other hand, cannot attack the germs directly, as streptomycin can. But just because they're changeable they can endlessly readjust to new circumstances and

285

assume new positions. Unless, of course, they become too explicit, or follow too rigid a program, in which case they become identical with science, sharing its inflexibility without being able to duplicate its practical effectiveness.

This was the risk the crusade's leaders ran, depriving their images of power by overmethodizing or scientizing them. When Bernarr MacFadden took generally current (and reputable) ideas about the wholesomeness of fresh air and pure food, codified these pleasantly unspecific theories into a rigid plan for dumbbell workouts, friction baths, and raw vegetables, he reduced them to demonstrable absurdity and threatened to discredit them. This, perhaps, is the root of the otherwise puzzling but apparently deliberate vagueness about consumption among the real professionals of imagery, the writers, like James and O'Neill. They knew an imaginative vision needed to be built up, but not too far. If it became too elaborate it lost its plasticity, hence its power to engage the mind in its irrational depths as well as on its reasonable surface. "Heaven forbid," James rather archly insists of Milly Theale, "we should 'know' anything more of our ravaged sister than what Densher darkly pieces together. . . . For we have time, while this passage lasts, to turn round critically; we have time to recognise intentions and proprieties; we have time to catch glimpses of an economy of composition, as I put it, interesting in itself. . . ." Imagination, rightly used, gives us time, and, James might have added, space.

Scientific knowledge doesn't, and in that sense it is not our most flexible ally against disease, though it has proved our most potent, when it works. When Robert Koch walked into his Berlin lecture hall on March 24, 1882, he was on the verge of announcing not merely a major breakthrough but a decisive turn in the way the West dealt with illness, though in the case of consumption the movement he began would take the better part of a century to complete itself. And in the meantime a middle way had to be found, amenable to the scientific method but also able to address the needs it could not yet satisfy. The result was bricolage—improvisation, an unsystematic appeal to all the currents of thought that might plausibly work against the disease without demeaning or ostracizing its victims. Science ruled, perhaps, but it was infiltrated by many other streams as well. In one of the subtler ironies of the era, the American Medical Association, meeting at St. Paul, Minnesota, in June of 1882, just three months after Koch's announcement, completely ignored it. Yet the keynote address by Dr. P. O. Hooper, was a fervent paean to the very science the association was in practice ignoring:

> The bounds of the horizon of investigation have been stretched out. The fierce light of truth has disclosed the harmless nature of many a veiled superstition. Much, regarded for centuries as but the dream of philosophers, has proven reality. Predictions never supposed to be aught but theories have been verified. The chains and bolts of formalism have been broken; and the devotees of science have pushed their explorations with audacious courage in every direction.

Science, yes, but not the tubercle bacillus. When Trudeau excitedly broke the news of Koch's discovery to his friend and already eminent mentor, Alfred Loomis, the latter laconically replied that he "didn't believe much in 'germs.'"

That reflects the looseness of thought that went under the heading of science early in the movement. And if it lacked rigor, it admitted a richness that left the cure as time went on and, at first through surgery and finally through antibiotics, both medicine in general and tuberculosis medicine in particular became more and more methodical, more and more empirical. The balance between imagination and science could not be, or at least was not, sustained. The mysteries vanished (or rather appeared to vanish), and the metaphors gave way.

In which something was lost. For though the themes of this last crusade may have distorted tuberculosis and may even at times have spread misinformation about it, they revealed other truths. They told us what we thought about our cities and our social relations with each other. They told us how we viewed our bodies, what we meant when we said "healthy" and "sick." As medicine fought itself clear of other professions and other disciplines, it also separated illness from the rest of lived life, thus depriving it of its power to reveal things to us. Sanatoriums were a comment on what Americans thought about the country, on what they saw as the ideal city, on the proper organization of an economy.

The first European Crusades to the Holy Land were, arguably, vain and cruel, the instigators of untold folly and suffering, but in them, battling against self-proclaimed enemies and testing themselves on foreign ground against an alien culture, Europeans began to define themselves, and that set the stage for growth and discovery. The War on Consumption, a modern and, to its proponents, a still more vital crusade, directed against a more formidable enemy, also perpetrated its incidental cruelties and follies. But as it deployed the human imagination against an immemorial terror, it achieved more than a clinical victory. For, as it engaged with the most mortal and most pervasive of all diseases, probing its causes, tracing our weakness before it and our occasional triumphs against it, it told us more than the truths of biology. It told us who we were.

Notes

Introduction

page

5: **another, more primitive story . . .**—My account of the
life cycle of *mycobacterium tuberculosis humanis* and
the history of its relations with mankind relies on the
following: G. P. Youmans, *Tuberculosis* (Philadelphia:
Saunders, 1979); René and Jean Dubos, *The White
Plague: Tuberculosis, Man and Society* (Boston: Little,
Brown, 1952); S. C. Robbins, R. S. Cotran, and V.
Kumar, *Pathologic Basis of Disease,* 3d ed.
(Philadelphia: Saunders, 1984); Wolfgang Joklik, Hilda
Willett, and D. Bernard Amos, eds., *Zinsser Microbi-
ology* (Norwalk, Conn.: Appleton-Century-Crofts,
1984); article on tuberculosis by John M. Grange, in
Topley and Wilson, *Principles of Bacteriology, Virol-
ogy, and Immunity,* vol. 3 (Baltimore: Williams and
Wilkins, 1984); article on mycobacteria by R. M. Des
Prez and R. A. Goodwin, Jr., in G. L. Mandell, R. G.
Douglas, Jr., and J. E. Bennett, *Principles and Practice*

of *Infectious Diseases,* 2d ed. (New York: Wiley, 1985); C. L. Erhardt and J. E. Berlin, eds., *Mortality and Morbidity in the United States* (Cambridge: Harvard University Press, 1974); P. F. Wehrle and F. H. Top, eds., *Communicable and Infectious Diseases* (St. Louis: Mosby, 1981).

Chapter One: "The Sorrow of the Cities": Images of Tuberculosis in the Nineteenth Century

page

16: "Never spent an hour . . ."—My account of Thoreau's last illness follows Henry S. Canby, *Thoreau* (Boston: Beacon Press, 1939), pp. 438–40.

17: "one of the mercifullest . . ."—Sir Thomas Browne, manuscript passage probably intended for the "Letter to a Friend," *The Works of Sir Thomas Browne,* ed. Geoffrey Keynes (Chicago: University of Chicago Press, 1964), 1:121.

18: "Only extreme illness . . ."—Quoted in Milton Meltzer and Walter Harding, *A Thoreau Profile* (New York: Crowell, 1962), p. 286.

18: "a damned rascal . . ."—Canby, op. cit., p. 211.

18: "why he was so disappointed, . . ."—Ibid., p. xix.

18: "I feel like saying . . ."—Meltzer and Harding, op. cit., p. 288.

19: "Few lives contain . . ."—*Atlantic Monthly,* August 1862, p. 240.

19: "There is a flower . . ."—Ibid., p. 249.

20: "most peculiar and baffling . . ."—Sidney Lanier, *Poems and Letters,* ed. Charles R. Anderson (Baltimore: Johns Hopkins University Press, 1969), Letter 7.

20: "Reverend Marsh, . . ."—Ibid., pp. 63–64.

21: "How dark, how dark . . ."—Ibid., p. 67.

22: Acquiring useless, or even harmful things . . .—See Thorstein Veblen, *Theory of the Leisure Class* (New York: B. W. Huebsch, 1922), pp. 68–101.

23: "In contrast to the diseases . . ."—Quoted in René and Jean Dubos, *The White Plague: Tuberculosis, Man and Society,* p. 53.

23: "Little Eliza had inherited, . . ."—Quoted in Richard H. Shryock, *National Tuberculosis Association, 1904–54: A Study of the Voluntary Health Movement in the United States* (New York: National Tuberculosis Association, 1957), p. 40.

23: "She was wasted . . ."—Ibid., p. 40.

24: "When Jo came home that spring, . . ."—Louisa M. Alcott, *Little Women* (New York: Modern Library, 1983), p. 456.

24: "in the dark hour . . ."—Ibid., p. 514.

25: "I discovered without difficulty . . ."—Alexandre Dumas *fils, The Lady of the Camellias,* tr. Edmund Gosse (New York: Collier, 1902), pp. 2–3.

26: "It was terrible to see, . . ."—Ibid., p. 60.

26: "The room to which she had fled . . ."—Ibid., p. 103.

26: " 'If I decide . . .' "—Ibid., p. 113.

27: "She had known nothing . . ."—Henri Murger, "Francine and Her Muff," *Bohemian Life,* tr. Leslie Orde (New York: Brentano's, 1901), p. 168.

27: "Bother the dead leaves, . . ."—Ibid., p. 168.

28: "Now a strange thing happened. . . ."—Ibid., p. 175.

30: "One lived on the old homestead, . . ."—Henry Bowditch, "Consumption in America," *Atlantic Monthly,* January 1869, p. 54.

30: "It is too cold, . . ."—Ibid., *Atlantic Monthly,* March 1869, p. 319.

31: "Little Jim, . . ."—Catharine E. Beecher and Harriet Beecher Stowe, *The American Woman's Home, or Principles of Domestic Science* (reprint ed., New York: Arno Press, 1971), p. 50.

32: "I myself, . . ."—J. H. Bennet, *On the Treatment of Pulmonary Consumption by Hygiene, Climate, and Medicine* (New York: Appleton, 1872), p. 37.

32: "the requirements of a suitable . . ."—William Osler,

The Principles and Practice of Medicine (New York: Appleton, 1892), pp. 250–51.

32: "I went from Edinburgh . . ."—Bennet, op. cit., pp. 148–49.

33: "The hearth-stone was really the gathering place . . ."—Bowditch, op. cit., *Atlantic Monthly*, February 1869, p. 179.

33: "Cities exercise a mysterious attraction . . ."—Bennet, op. cit., p. 135.

34: "Scene 5—A court . . ."—*Monthly Confidential Bulletin of the Work of Anti-Tuberculosis Associations*, mimeographed, August 1913, p. 2.

34: " 'And now we come to the other side . . .' "—Ibid., p. 4.

35: "instruction in precautions necessary . . ."—John C. Gebhart, *Tuberculosis, A Family Problem: The Story of the Home Hospital of the A.I.C.P.* (New York: New York Association for Improving the Condition of the Poor, 1924), pp. 5–6.

36: "At the present time . . ."—Bowditch, op. cit., *Atlantic Monthly*, February 1869, p. 181.

36: "Viewed in this light, . . ."—Bennet, op. cit., p. 17.

36: "We have seen cases where mental suffering, . . ." —Bowditch, op. cit., *Atlantic Monthly*, February 1869, p. 185.

36: "While requiring absolute attention . . ."—Ibid., *Atlantic Monthly*, March 1869, p. 322.

37: "The era of science . . ."—Mary Baker Glover (Eddy), *Science and Health* (Boston: Christian Scientist Publishing Co., 1875), p. 116.

38: "Why . . . cannot we all throw trouble off . . ."—*Mount McGregor Optimist*, Early Spring 1938, p. 26.

38: "If you must be blue, . . ."—Betty MacDonald, *The Plague and I* (Philadelphia: Lippincott, 1948), p. 57.

39: All had a few mild herbs . . .—See A. Emil Hiss, *Thesaurus of Proprietary Preparations and Pharmaceutical Specialties* (Chicago: G. P. Engelhard, 1899), pp. 223, 228, and 239.

Chapter Two: "The Greatest Battle Ever Fought": Edward Livingston Trudeau and the War on Consumption

page

40: "as nearly everybody had malaria . . ."—Edward Livingston Trudeau, *An Autobiography* (Garden City, N.Y.: Doubleday Page, 1916), p. 70.

41: " 'Well, Dr. Janeway, . . .' "—Ibid., pp. 71–72.

41: a dull sound when one tapped the chest . . .—See Osler, *The Principles and Practice of Medicine*, p. 226.

42: "During the entire journey . . ."—Trudeau, op. cit., p. 80.

44: "From childhood he had been delicate, . . ."—Ibid., p. 29.

44: "I have had ample opportunity . . ."—Ibid., p. 74.

46: "Bring out your individual qualities. . . ."—Charlie Porth, in the *Mount McGregor Optimist,* Early Spring 1938, p. 7.

46: "On several occasions I have been taken . . ."—Trudeau, op. cit., pp. 97–98.

47: "As I lay comfortably . . ."—Ibid., pp. 87–88.

48: "Many a beautiful afternoon . . ."—Ibid., p. 165–66.

49: "The mountains now look down . . ."—Ibid., p. 172.

50: His grandson, Dr. Francis Trudeau, compares his state of mind . . .—Interview, August 1986.

52: by 1901 there were eight statewide associations . . .—See Shryock, *National Tuberculosis Association, 1904–54,* pp. 54–55.

52: "I cannot find words . . ."—Quoted in ibid., p. 77.

53: "Dodgers are distributed . . ."—*Confidential Bulletin,* December 1908, p. 3.

54: "Find a busy man . . ."—Ibid.

54: "along lines somewhat similar . . ."—*Confidential Bulletin,* February 1909, p. 6.

54: "black pins indicate . . ."—Ibid., p. 7.

54: "a determined crusade . . ."—*Confidential Bulletin,* December 1908, p. 5.

54: "DON'T SPIT on the floor . . ."—Quoted in *Confidential Bulletin,* January 1909, p. 10.

55: "THE AMUSEMENT PROBLEM . . ."—*Confidential Bulletin,* November 1912, p. 7.

56: "a Miss Mary Rossiter . . ."—*Confidential Bulletin,* January 1913, p. 2.

56: All arms of the cross were to be pointed; . . .—*Confidential Bulletin,* September 1913, p. 3.

57: "This crusade against the Great White Plague . . ." —*Confidential Bulletin,* July 1914, p. 6. The crusade was, of course, allied (though informally) to the Progressive movement. See Richard Hofstadter, *The Age of Reform* (New York: Knopf, 1955).

57: "Neither prosperity, nor its consequent power to achieve . . ."—*The Dedication of the Metropolitan Life Insurance Company's Tuberculosis Sanatorium* (Mt. McGregor, N.Y.: Metropolitan Life Insurance Company, 1914), p. 13.

60: "We must confess the sad and unwelcome truth . . ." —Bowditch, op. cit., *Atlantic Monthly,* January 1869, p. 56.

62: "I've been with the painters of rainbows, . . ." —George M. P. Baird, "The Theft of Thistledown," *Journal of the Outdoor Life,* November 1915, p. 348.

62: "All alone in a grimy basket, . . ."—Ibid., p. 349.

62: "When the baby cried . . ."—Ibid.

62: "The world growing better, mankind . . ."—Ibid., pp. 349–50.

63: "And you, O people of the earth, . . ."—Ibid., p. 350.

64: "O, sister life, . . ."—George M. P. Baird, "The Narrow Door," *Journal of the Outdoor Life,* November 1915, pp. 350–51.

64: "ignorance of the wise, . . ."—Ibid., p. 351.

64: "O women who spin, have you seen . . ."—Ibid., p. 352.

64: "Mankind, not Death, . . ."—Ibid., pp. 352–53.

65: "O men and children of men, . . ."—Ibid., p. 353.

Notes

66: "sickness, sin and death . . ."—Mary Baker Glover (Eddy), *Science and Health*, p. 116.

Chapter Three: "Rules and a Daily Routine": The Rise of the Sanatorium

page

68: "a huge Gothic pile, . . ."—F. Rufenacht Walters, *Sanatoria for Consumptives: A Critical and Detailed Description* (London: Swan Sonnenschein, 1902), p. 151.

68: "a murmuring rivulet of crystal purity . . ."—Reinhard Ortmann, *Görbersdorf, Dr. Brehmer's Sanatorium for Consumptives* (Zurich: Illustrated Europe Series, Fussli, 188[?]), p. 21.

68: "We are irresistibly reminded . . ."—Ibid., p. 21.

69: "useful maxims"—Walters, op. cit., p. 151.

69: "naturally varying in size . . ."—Ortmann, op. cit., pp. 31–32.

70: "felt in the blood, . . ."—William Wordsworth, "Lines Composed a Few Miles above Tintern Abbey," *The Poetical Works of Wordsworth*, ed. Thomas Hutchinson and Ernest de Selincourt (London: Oxford University Press, 1960), p. 164.

72: "The region has no population able . . ."—J. J. Duryea, in Joseph W. Stickler, M.D., *The Adirondacks as a Health Resort* (New York: Putnam's, 1886), pp. 51–52.

73: "I began to wonder how, . . ."—Quoted in Gordon M. Meade, M.D., "Edward Livingston Trudeau, M.D.," *Tubercle* (1972), p. 238.

73n: The Channing Home . . .—See Julius Wilson, M.D., "Trudeau and Before Trudeau" (MS, unpub.), and "Early Tuberculosis Sanatoria in the United States" (MS, unpub., 1968).

74: had become resident physician . . .—See Edward Livingston Trudeau, *An Autobiography*, pp. 285–86.

74: "He's swell"—Marshall McClintock, *We Take to Bed*

(New York: Jonathan Cape and Harrison Smith, 1931), p. 109.

75: **an inventor, among other things, . . .**—See S. Adolphus Knopf, *Tuberculosis as a Disease of the Masses and How to Combat It,* 5th ed. (facsimile reprint, New York: Arno Press, 1977), p. 94.

76: **" 'unfaithful to the cure'. . ."**—Lawrason Brown, *Rules for Recovery from Pulmonary Tuberculosis,* 2d ed. (Philadelphia: Lea and Febiger, 1916), p. 64.

76: **"Patients must spend . . ."**—F. Rufenacht Walters, op. cit., p. 498.

76: **"It is surprising . . ."**—Knopf, op. cit., pp. 67–68.

77: **"Plush velvet or cloth . . ."**—Ibid., p. 24.

78: **"should face south . . ."**—Lawrason Brown, op. cit., p. 72.

78: **"Place the rug, . . ."**—Ibid., p. 74.

79: **"7:30 . . ."**—Ibid., pp. 61–62.

80: **Knopf thought forty degrees . . .**—See Knopf, op. cit., p. 34.

81: **Thomas S. Carrington . . .**—See Thomas S. Carrington, M.D., *Tuberculosis Hospital and Sanatorium Construction,* 3d. ed. (New York: National Association for the Study and Prevention of Tuberculosis, 1914), p. 37.

81: **"It is an old adage . . ."**—Lawrason Brown, op. cit., p. 44.

82: **Charles Fox Gardiner, . . .**—Dietary details and quotations following are from Charles Fox Gardiner, M.D., *The Care of the Consumptive* (New York: Putnam's, 1900), pp. 44–49.

83: **even O'Neill's stage directions . . .**—See Eugene O'Neill, *The Straw,* in *The Plays of Eugene O'Neill* (New York: Random House, 1928), 3:375–76.

84: **"Rest," according to the Metropolitan Life . . .**—See *Instructions and Information for Patients* (Mount McGregor, N.Y.: Metropolitan Life Insurance Company Sanatorium, 1942), pp. 5–8.

84: *"Some Aphorisms for the Tuberculosis Patient . . ."* —Edward O. Otis, M.D., *The Great White Plague Tuberculosis* (New York: Crowell, 1909), p. 141.

85: "A slight feeling of lassitude, . . ."—Lawrason Brown, op. cit., p. 91.

86: "a school, a college . . ."—S. Adolphus Knopf, "The Ideal Sanatorium, the Ideal Physician, the Ideal Nurse, the Ideal Patient," *New York Medical Journal*, 18 October 1919, p. 9.

86: "I wish Dr. Fishberg . . ."—Ibid., p. 12.

86: "the constant and continuous exposure . . ."—Edward O. Otis, op. cit., p. 106.

86: "Tranquillity and hopefulness of mind, . . ."—Ibid., p. 107.

87: "Consumption is curable . . ."—M. J. Brooks, M.D., *Gleanings from Twelve Years' Constant Residence in a Sanatorium for the Treatment of Pulmonary Tuberculosis* (New York: Privately printed, 1908), p. 16.

87: "It may . . . be said . . ."—Carrington, op. cit., p. 1.

88: Carrington estimated that in 1914 . . .—Ibid., p. 13f.

89: "constructed of substantial material . . ."—Ibid., p. 36.

89: A typical example . . .—Ibid., p. 24.

89n: the design for the Georgia State Sanatorium . . .—Ibid., p. 25.

91: by 1935 there were, . . .—See Council on Medical Education and Hospitals of the American Medical Association, "Survey of Tuberculosis Hospitals and Sanatoriums in the United States," *Journal of the American Medical Association*, 7 December 1935, p. 1857.

92: Early in its history . . .—Alexis de Tocqueville, *Democracy in America*, tr. Henry Reeve, ed. Francis Bowen and Phillips Bradley (New York: Vintage, 1945), 2: 114–22.

92: "the beginning of a broad movement . . ."—Quoted in *The Loomis Sanatorium for the Treatment of Tuberculosis: An Account of Its Origin, Foundation and*

Development (Loomis, N.Y.: Loomis Sanatorium, 1921), pp. 43–44.

92: "The building of this cottage . . ."—Ibid., pp. 50–52.

93: "this class of institution . . ."—Carrington, op. cit., p. 12.

93: "As it is undesirable . . ."—Walters, op. cit., p. 27.

94: "light carpentering, . . ."—Carrington, op. cit., p. 41.

94: "The sanatorium has a great . . ."—Ibid., p. 22.

95: John Humphrey Noyes, . . .—See Maren L. Carden, *Oneida: Utopian Community to Modern Corporation* (Baltimore: Johns Hopkins University Press, 1969).

95: The Chautauqua movement, . . .—See J. E. Gould, *The Chautauqua Movement: An Episode in the Continuing American Revolution* (Albany: State University of New York Press, 1961).

Chapter Four: "Our Serene Life": Rituals of the Cure

page

98: "NOTICE TO ACCEPTED CANDIDATES . . ."—W. L. Rathbun, M.D., *The Municipal Sanatorium at Otisville,* 2d ed. (New York: Department of Health, 1914), p. 27.

99: In the Middle Ages, . . .—See George Rosen, *A History of Public Health* (New York: MD Publications, 1958), pp. 64–65.

100: "The living and dressing rooms . . ."—Rathbun, op. cit., pp. 16–17.

101: "Your chances of getting well . . ."—Ibid., pp. 34–35.

102: The "sick role," . . .—See Talcott Parsons, *On Institutions and Social Evolution,* ed. Leon H. Mayhew (Chicago: University of Chicago Press, 1982), pp. 149–51.

102: "My first glimpse . . ."—Henry Levy, writing in the *Ray Brook Oracle* [New York State Archives], July 1954, n.p.

103: "The ride from the station . . ."—Ibid.

104: "A smiling buxom woman . . ."—Isabel Smith, *Wish I Might* (New York: Harper and Row, 1955), p. 28.

104: "The room, with its pale painted walls . . ."—Ibid., p. 70.

105: "as my bed neared the windows, . . ."—Ibid., p. 71.

106: "If you want to cure in the kind of a San . . ."—Quoted in *Journal of the Outdoor Life,* October 1920, p. 278.

107: "From that time on . . ."—Isabel Smith, op. cit., p. 177.

107: "It would be my Trouble Book . . ."—Ibid., p. 62.

108: "Writing in my Trouble Book . . ."—Ibid.

108: "When the porch was ready . . ."—Clara N. Bates, "It Can Be Done," *Journal of the Outdoor Life,* July 1920, p. 199.

108: "Her friends . . ."—Ibid., pp. 199–200.

109: In transit to his sanatorium, . . .—Alan Dick, *Walking Miracle* (London: Allen and Unwin, 1942), p. 21.

109: "Beside me was the farmer's son . . ."—Ibid., p. 57.

109: "You went into hospital a sick man . . ."—Ibid., p. 123.

110: "We entered the Pines . . ."—Betty MacDonald, *The Plague and I,* pp. 49–50.

110: "The waiting room . . ."—Ibid., pp. 51–52.

111: "Really one doesn't have as much time . . ."—Sadie Fuller Seagrave, *Saints Rest* (St. Louis: Mosby, 1918), pp. 59–60.

112: "I had to remind myself . . ."—Betty MacDonald, op. cit., p. 75.

112: "IF YOU HAVE NOTHING TO DO, . . ."—Ibid., p. 40.

112: "IF YOU THINK RIGHT, . . ."—Ibid., p. 122.

113: "Are you really in earnest . . ."—*Journal of the Outdoor Life,* November 1930, p. 658.

113: " 'I'm going to be married!' . . ."—Isabel Smith, op. cit., p. 187.

113: " 'All right, Izzy, dear,' . . ."—Ibid., p. 202.

113-4: "Trudeau's lovely little chapel . . ."—Ibid., p. 203.

114: "I always take the word of my nurses . . ."—Sadie Fuller Seagrave, op. cit., pp. 128–29.

114: "He doesn't set himself up like an autocrat, . . ." —Ibid., p. 143.

114: "To me Death is a lecherous, . . ."—Betty MacDonald, op. cit., p. 160.

115: "I awoke in the cold, . . ."—Ibid., pp. 171–72.

116: Yet her most specific memory . . .—Ruth Stern, Interview, March 1986.

116: nearly 25 percent of all patients died . . .—See Shryock, *National Tuberculosis Association, 1904–54,* p. 155.

117: "with a rule book, . . ."—Marshall McClintock, *We Take to Bed,* p. 126.

118: "From a purely practical point of view . . ."—Marian Spitzer, *I Took It Lying Down* (New York: Random House, 1951), p. 17.

118: "Pretty nearly all TB patients . . ."—Ibid., p. 22.

118: "You *have* an enemy, . . ."—Ibid.

118: "The language of the sanatorium is unique . . ."—John Potts, *Getting Well and Staying Well: A Book for Tuberculous Patients, Public Health Nurses, and Doctors* (St. Louis: Mosby, 1927), p. 105.

119: "They say to their medical attendant: . . ."—Ibid.

119: "These patients . . ."—Ibid.

119: "A chart is rather like a lie detector, . . ."—Marian Spitzer, op. cit., p. 67.

120: a 1925 program . . .—*Graduation Exercises: The Graduates of the September Class of 1925,* souvenir program (Saranac Lake, N.Y.: Trudeau Sanatorium, 1925), n.p.

121: "tooling and putting together wallets, . . ."—Isabel Smith, op. cit., pp. 83–84.

122: "a crocheted napkin ring, . . ."—Betty MacDonald, op. cit., p. 219.

123: "You're no better . . ."—Ibid., p. 238.

124: "I love to lie on my sleeping porch . . ."—Laura Rose Underhill, *Journal of the Outdoor Life,* September 1928, p. 553.

124: In 1955 the Firland Sanatorium . . .—See Catherine E. Vavra and Edith D. Rainboth, *A Study of Patients' Attitudes Toward Care at Firland Sanatorium, Seattle, Washington* (Seattle: Firland Sanatorium, 1955).

125: "I felt there was a certain arrogance . . ."—Allan Seager, *A Frieze of Girls* (New York: McGraw-Hill, 1964), p. 227.

Chapter Five: "The Burden of Human Misery, Not Its Own": Saranac Lake

page

127: In January of 1920, . . .—Details of the festivities are drawn from the official program of the Mid-Winter Carnival, Saranac Lake, N.Y., 1920.

128: One year, . . .—See Philip L. Gallos, *Cure Cottages of Saranac Lake* (Saranac Lake, N.Y.: Historic Saranac Lake, 1985), illustration, p. 169.

129: Dr. Francis B. Trudeau could, . . .—Dr. Francis Trudeau, Interview, August 1986.

130: "I know now, . . ."—Marshall McClintock, *We Take to Bed*, p. 24.

130: "It is a big room . . ."—Elizabeth Mooney, *In the Shadow of the White Plague* (New York: Crowell, 1979), p. 11.

131: "A number of episodes . . ."—*Adirondack Enterprise,* 28 October 1925.

131: "wonderful, . . . beautiful."—Esther Mirick, Oral history tape, interview by Philip L. Gallos (Saranac Lake, N.Y.: Saranac Lake Free Library, 1982).

131: "as much fun there"—Bill McLaughlin, Oral history tape, interview by Philip L. Gallos (Saranac Lake, N.Y.: Saranac Lake Free Library, 1982).

131: "no duds . . ."—Ibid.

132: "completely run for the sick people";—Esther Mirick, Oral history tape, interview by Philip L. Gallos, cited above.

132: Its story was, . . .—For Saranac's early history, see Henry W. Raymond, *The Story of Saranac: A Chapter in Adirondack History* (New York: Grafton Publishers, 1909). The town's official name is Saranac Lake.

Though it is often called "Saranac" for short, this occasions some confusion, since there is a small village by that name in Clinton County, about thirty-five miles northeast of Saranac Lake.

132: **"When [Smith] came into the Adirondacks . . ."** —Francis Trudeau, "Saranac Lake and Tuberculosis," baccalaureate thesis, Yale College, on deposit at Saranac Lake Free Library.

133: **"The Adirondack Mountains, as Dr. Trudeau found them, . . ."**—*Adirondack Enterprise,* 15 November 1915.

133: **"Here . . . there is every inducement . . ."**—Alfred Loomis, M.D., "The Adirondack Region as a Therapeutic Agent in the Treatment of Pulmonary Tuberculosis," *Medical Record,* 26 April 1879, p. 386.

134: **"My sister and I were assigned to the 'Little Red'** . . ."—Carolyn Pentland Lindsay, MS memoir solicited for 1925 anniversary issue of the *Journal of the Outdoor Life,* in archives of Trudeau Institute, Saranac Lake, N.Y. (file 1050).

134-5: **"sat shut up in a glass cabinet . . ."**—Ibid.

135: **"For nine months I had daily injections . . ."**—Emeline Cooper, MS memoir solicited for 1925 anniversary issue of the *Journal of the Outdoor Life,* in archives of Trudeau Institute, Saranac Lake, N.Y. (file 1050).

135: **"There are about 100 invalids . . ."**—*New York Evening Post,* 19 March 1898.

138: **Adelaide Crapsey's cure cottage . . .**—See Robert Taylor, *Saranac: America's Magic Mountain* (Boston: Houghton Mifflin, 1986), p. 125f. Taylor's book offers lively accounts of the celebrities who lived in or passed through Saranac during the heyday of the cure.

139: **"Situated on the summit of Helen Street Hill . . ."** —Advertisement, Carnival Edition, *Northern New Yorker,* 1907.

139: **Phil Gallos . . .**—See Philip L. Gallos, *Cure Cottages of Saranac Lake,* pp. 53–57.

140: **"Slightly delayed on their scheduled automobile trip . . ."**—*Adirondack Enterprise,* 16 July 1926.

141: **Invalids were listed . . .**—Sources for this and following statistics are the Adirondack directories and Saranac Lake telephone directories for the years cited.

143: **"Health-seekers feel . . ."**—Untitled brochure, ca. 1945, in archives of Trudeau Institute, Saranac Lake, N.Y. (file 1138).

143: **"MARCELLING *as it should be done,* . . ."**—Advertisement, *Jubilee Book in Commemoration of the Fifth Anniversary of the Hospitalization at Saranac Lake, New York, of Disabled Veterans of the World War* (Saranac Lake, N.Y., ca. 1925).

144: **"The Saranac Lake Society . . ."**—Quoted in Philip L. Gallos, *Cure Cottages of Saranac Lake,* pp. 16–17.

144: **a list of boarding cottages . . .**—Ibid., p. 17.

144: **"My own idea . . ."**—E. R. Baldwin, M.D., MS letter in archives of Trudeau Institute, Saranac Lake, N.Y. (file 1141).

145: **"clearly one of an accidental nature, . . ."**—*Northern New Yorker,* 16 January 1907.

145: **a famous 1930 incident . . .**—See, for example, Elizabeth Mooney, op. cit., p. 75.

145: **"Being told we have tuberculosis, . . ."**—*Regain Your Health in Saranac Lake* [promotional pamphlet] (Saranac Lake, N.Y., 1935).

145: **"poor suffering mortals . . ."**—Quoted in *Adirondack Enterprise,* 14 July 1926.

145: **"How little those who so often speak . . ."**—Edward Livingston Trudeau, *An Autobiography,* p. 316.

147: **"Saranac Lake is a closely built village. . . ."**—Forrest B. Ames, "A Tuberculosis Survey of the Residents of Saranac Lake, New York," *American Review of Tuberculosis,* June 1918, p. 217.

149: **"Everything was humming right along . . ."**—Bill

McLaughlin, Oral history tape, interview by Philip L. Gallos, cited above.

149: **Perhaps nothing brackets the rise and fall . . .**—Statistics and quotations following are from Mary Prescott's *Annual Report* on the Reception Hospital, issued yearly from 1902 until 1949, privately printed, and on deposit at the Saranac Lake Free Library, Saranac Lake, N.Y.

Chapter Six: "Fewer and Better Doctors": Tuberculosis and the Medical Profession

page

152: **In 1850 the United States had fifty-two medical schools; . . .**—See Paul Starr, *The Social Transformation of American Medicine* (New York: Basic Books, 1982), p. 112.

153: **"There was no entrance examination. . . ."**—Edward Livingston Trudeau, *An Autobiography,* pp. 37–38.

154: **On that day one Stewart McMurtry . . .**—Material on McMurtry's case is from Francis Delafield's notebook on respiratory cases, on deposit at the New York Academy of Medicine.

155: **"an association in which there will be no medical politics . . ."**—Quoted in Paul Starr, op. cit., p. 91.

155: **intermittent pains . . .**—Delafield, notebook, p. 6.

156: **a number of tubercles, . . .**—Ibid., p. 29.

156: **Rather Virchow saw pathology . . .**—See William R. Coleman, *Biology in the Nineteenth Century: Problems of Form, Function and Transformation* (New York: Wiley, 1971), p. 32; and John P. Dolan and W. N. Adams-Smith, *A Documentary History of Medicine* (New York: Seabury Press, 1978), pp. 141–42.

158: **Koch, born in the Harz Mountains . . .**—See Grace T. Hallock and C. E. Turner, *Robert Koch* (New York: Metropolitan Life Insurance Company, Health Heroes Series, 1932).

158: "surviving mainly . . ."—Ibid., pp. 3–4.

158: "had no love . . ."—Ibid., p. 6.

159: "Drop everything . . ."—Ibid., p. 15.

160: "Tuberculosis has so far been . . ."—Robert Koch, "The Aetiology of Tuberculosis," tr. Berna and Max Pinner, *American Review of Tuberculosis,* March 1932, p. 322.

160: "No other single physician's work . . ."—Allen K. Krause, Introduction to "The Aetiology of Tuberculosis," *American Review of Tuberculosis,* March 1932, p. 293.

161: "Koch has ascertained . . ."—*New York World,* 23 April 1882.

161: "An ardent believer . . ."—*New York Times,* 5 May 1882.

162: Koch, loath to disappoint, . . .—See René and Jean Dubos, *The White Plague: Tuberculosis, Man and Society,* p. 104f.

163: "a clear, brownish liquid, . . ."—Robert Koch, *The Cure of Consumption: Further Communications on a Remedy for Tuberculosis,* tr. anon. (London: Heinemann, 1890), p. 6.

163: "Three or four hours after the injection . . ."—Ibid., pp. 9–10.

164: "It will be quite possible . . ."—Ibid., p. 17.

164: In the excitement, his younger sister died . . .—*Review of Reviews,* December 1890, p. 551.

164: Sir Arthur Conan Doyle, . . .—See ibid., p. 556.

165: By 1891, 2,172 consumptives had been treated . . . —*Journal of the American Medical Association,* 23 May 1891, p. 745.

165-6: "a glycerine extract . . ."—Robert Koch, "Additional Communications Concerning a Remedy for Tuberculosis," tr. Paul Ehrlich, *Journal of the American Medical Association,* 21 February 1891, pp. 262–65.

166: "the hands of swindlers."—*Review of Reviews,* December 1890, p. 551.

166: "had come to an agreement . . ."—Ibid., p. 551.

166: "my work is not yet completed"—Koch, *The Cure of Consumption,* p. 5.

166: "of a somewhat disquieting character . . ."—Quoted in *Journal of the American Medical Association,* 7 February 1891, p. 206.

167: "Dr. Koch's remedy . . ."—*Journal of the American Medical Association,* 21 February 1891, p. 286.

168: "Twenty years ago, . . ."—Quoted in *Review of Reviews,* April 1891, p. 369.

168: Guiseppe [*sic*] Arnoldi, . . .—Delafield, notebook, p. 34.

170: "is confronted by a definite situation . . ."—Abraham Flexner, *Medical Education in the United States and Canada: A Report to the Carnegie Foundation for the Advancement of Teaching* (New York: Carnegie Foundation, 1910), p. 53.

172: "The improvement of medical education . . ."—Ibid., pp. 16–17.

173: "The medical profession is a social organ, . . ."—Ibid., p. 42.

173: "with the advent of the laboratory, . . ."—Ibid., p. 22.

174: a control over the conditions of work . . .—See, for example, Eliot L. Freidson, *Profession of Medicine: A Study of the Sociology of Applied Knowledge* (New York: Dodd Mead, 1970), pp. 71–84.

174: Magali Sarfatti Larson, . . .—See Magali Sarfatti Larson, *The Rise of Professionalism: A Sociological Analysis* (Berkeley: University of California Press, 1977), chapter 2.

175: "means that escape rules . . ."—H. Jamous and B. Peloille, quoted in ibid., p. 42.

175: consistently emphasize the indeterminacy of it, . . .—See Eliot L. Freidson, op. cit., p. 169f.

175: "like political or economic power, . . ."—Ibid., p. 170.

177: In a report to the city health department, . . .—See Shryock, *National Tuberculosis Association, 1904–54,* p. 50.

177: "the discovery of the possibilities . . ."—Quoted in ibid., p. 56.

Chapter Seven: "Plainly Designed for the Public Good": Reform, Philanthropy, and Business

page

179: *"Luft—luft—gib mir luft"*—Ernest Poole, *The Plague in Its Stronghold* (New York: Committee on the Prevention of Tuberculosis of the Charity Organization Society of the City of New York, 1903), p. 3.

180: Even in 1903, . . .—Ibid., p. 7.

182: he actually set the place on fire . . .—See Jacob A. Riis, *How the Other Half Lives: Studies among the Tenements of New York* (reprint ed., New York: Dover, 1971), p. 30.

183: "Bottle Alley . . . is a fair specimen . . ."—Ibid., p. 54.

184: "It is a Plague in disguise. . . ."—Poole, op. cit., pp. 4–5.

185: "The court looks like a deep pit; . . ."—Ibid., p. 15.

186: "wilfully careless consumptives . . ."—C. E. A. Winslow, *The Life of Hermann M. Biggs* (Philadelphia: Lea and Febiger, 1929), p. 190.

186: pleading but doomed, . . .—See Edwin S. Brown, *The House of Strength* (Boston: Four Seas Company, 1922), p. 24.

186: "It's got to come anyway, . . ."—Poole, op. cit., p. 21.

186: "I must keep my skin clean, . . ."—Riis, op. cit., p. 91.

187: Biggs and his father used to execute contracts . . .—See Winslow, op. cit., p. 22. My account of Biggs's life generally follows Winslow's exhaustively documented biography.

187: "Upon the recognition . . ."—Ibid., p. 40.

189: "Do not fail . . ."—Ibid., p. 88.

189: "It shall be the duty . . ."—Ibid., p. 132.

190: "The Board of Health formally declared war . . ."—*New York Sun*, 15 February 1894.

190: "If as many deaths . . ."—Winslow, op. cit., p. 138.

191: "The real obnoxiousness . . ."—Quoted in ibid., p. 144.

191: "it is . . . the extra missionary work . . ."—Quoted in ibid., p. 146.

192: "greatly exaggerated."—Ibid., p. 150.

192: "The government of the United States is democratic, . . ."—Ibid., p. 158.

192: "The most autocratic powers, . . ."—Ibid.

193: "as a means of avoiding the cultivation of habits of idleness . . ."—Ibid., p. 197.

193: "There were individuals . . ."—Ibid., p. 198.

194-5: not from the authority's ability to compel . . .—See, for example, Richard Sennett, *Authority* (New York: Knopf, 1980), p. 43.

196: "Americans of all ages, . . ."—De Tocqueville, *Democracy in America,* 2: 114.

197: The Framingham experiment . . .—My account of the demonstration relies on the most complete set of documents, the *Framingham Monographs,* a series of ten pamphlets, compiled and published by the Framingham Community Health Station between 1918 and 1924.

197: "the cooperation of local and state health officers, . . ."—*Framingham Monographs,* no. 1, p. 10.

197: "How . . . can social forces . . ."—Ibid., p. 11.

198: "an Exclusion Committee . . ."—Ibid., p. 16.

198: "neighborhood committees, . . ."—Ibid.

198: "light must be thrown, . . ."—Ibid., p. 20.

199: "insurance agents from the several larger companies"—Ibid., p. 19.

199: *"the first 500 Framingham families . . ."*—*Framingham Monographs,* no. 4, p. 45.

200: "You may find that while a family . . ."—Ibid., p. 43.

200: "popularly worded medical . . ."—Ibid., p. 8.

200: "nursing visits, . . ."—Ibid., p. 9.

201: Every Framingham consumptive was identified by a pin . . .—See *Framingham Monographs,* no. 5, p. 8.

201: The schools were found wanting . . .—See *Framing-*

ham Monographs, no. 6, p. 12. According to the reporting committee, 911 pupils, or 64.5 percent of the total surveyed, "were not fitted by their furniture in one or more ways."

202: "exposed to tuberculous infection . . ."—*Framingham Monographs,* no. 7, p. 9.

202: "Habits . . . Bathes weekly . . ."—Ibid., p. 31.

203: "Your Annual Medical Examination!! . . ."—*Framingham Monographs,* no. 8, p. 21.

204: "In this work the psychological appeals . . ."—*Framingham Monographs,* no. 10, p. 96.

205: "to make an owl weep . . ."—C. E. A. Winslow, *A City Set on a Hill: The Significance of the Health Demonstration at Syracuse, N.Y.* (New York: Doubleday, 1934), p. 16.

205: the tuberculosis death rate plummeted significantly . . .—Ibid., p. 155.

206: In 1904 the United States Senate . . .—See James Harvey Young, *The Medical Messiahs: A Social History of Health Quackery in Twentieth Century America* (Princeton: Princeton University Press, 1967), p. 68.

206: "Tubercleicide"—Ibid., p. 86.

206: "White Plague Conquered!!! . . ."—Ibid., p. 90.

208: " 'Died o' consumption, . . .' "—Clement Wood, *Bernarr MacFadden: A Study in Success* (New York: Lewis Copeland Co., 1929), p. 35.

208: "Bernarr MacFadden/Kinisitherapist . . ."—Ibid., p. 65.

209: "Seven A.M. Wake up! . . ."—Mary MacFadden and Emile Gauvreau, *Dumbbells and Carrot Strips* (London: Gollancz, 1956), pp. 11–12.

210: "Weakness is a crime. . . ."—Clement Wood, op. cit., p. 88.

210: "a form of vigorous massage"—MacFadden and Gauvreau, op. cit., p. 51.

210: "Pants in bed . . ."—Ibid., p. 3.

211: a course of walking on one's knees . . .—Ibid., p. 226.

211: "The victims of this terrible malady . . ."—Bernarr MacFadden, "Strengthening Weak Lungs—Curing Consumption: Vitality Building through Psycultopathy," (five-article series), article 1, *Physical Culture,* March 1909?, p. 206.

211: "vital resistance"—Ibid., p. 204.

212: "it is impossible . . ."—Ibid., article 2, *Physical Culture,* April 1909, p. 286.

212: "with every draught of air . . ."—Ibid., p. 286.

212: "Coffee, and tea, . . ."—Ibid., p. 289.

212: "it is much better . . ."—Ibid., article 5, *Physical Culture,* July 1909, p. 49.

212: "Don't worry . . ."—Ibid., p. 54.

213: *"No disease . . ."—Physical Culture,* September 1909, p. 279.

213: Linda Burfield, D.O., . . .—*Physical Culture,* December 1920, p. 44.

213: "Side view of a fat man, . . ."—*Physical Culture,* April 1909, p. 303.

214: "He is against the city, . . ."—Clement Wood, op. cit., pp. 292–93.

Chapter Eight: "Some Vague, Awful Thing": Novels, Plays, and Films

page

216: coughs, which he attributes to . . . shoe polish.—*Midnight Cowboy,* directed by John Schlesinger, screenplay by Waldo Salt (United Artists, 1969).

216: "Joe wanted to call it . . ."—James Leo Herlihy, *Midnight Cowboy* (New York: Dell, 1965), p. 155.

218: "Why . . . had one to look so straight . . ."—Henry James, *The Wings of the Dove,* ed. J. Donald Crowley and Richard A. Hocks (New York: Norton, 1978), p. 4.

218: "fall somehow into some abysmal trap . . ."—Ibid., p. 6.

218: "It would be of the essence . . ."—Ibid., p. 7.

219: "Heaven forbid, . . ."—Ibid., p. 12.

219: "imparting . . . to patches . . ."—Ibid., p. 13.

219: "he had . . . , with everyone else, . . ."—Ibid., p. 347.

220: "she can hardly be dying . . ."—F. O. Matthiessen, *Henry James: The Major Phase* (New York: Oxford University Press, 1963), p. 67.

220: " 'You're not loved enough.' . . ."—James, op. cit., p. 271.

220: " 'You'll come?' . . ."—Ibid., p. 312.

220: " 'Shall I at any rate suffer?' . . ."—Ibid., p. 151.

221: "in a state of uplifted . . ."—Ibid., p. 87.

221: "The romance for her, . . ."—Ibid., p. 266.

222: " 'Is it a bad case of lungs?' . . ."—Ibid., p. 214.

223: "For two very happy persons . . ."—Henry James, *The Ambassadors* (London: Everyman's Library, 1966), p. 328.

223: "Toward the end, . . ."—Quoted in Leon Edel, *Henry James: The Middle Years, 1882–1895* (New York: Avon, 1978), p. 302.

224: "I had absolute conviction . . ."—James, preface to *The Ambassadors,* quoted in *The Wings of the Dove,* p. 460.

225: "It is always difficult . . ."—James, *Notes of a Son and Brother,* quoted in *The Wings of the Dove,* p. 468.

226: "a brilliant boy, . . ."—Quoted in Arthur and Barbara Gelb, *O'Neill* (New York: Harper and Row, 1962), p. 216.

227: **44 percent of Gaylord Farm's discharged patients** . . .—See Shryock, *National Tuberculosis Association, 1904–54,* p. 155.

227: "It was at Gaylord . . ."—Quoted in Gelb, op. cit., p. 231.

228: "My blessings on the Farm . . ."—Ibid., p. 235.

229: "MRS. TURNER . . ."—O'Neill, *The Straw,* in *The Plays of Eugene O'Neill,* 3: 377–78.

229: "She must marry me at once . . ."—Ibid., p. 415.

231: "The right way is to remember"—Eugene O'Neill,

Long Day's Journey Into Night (New Haven: Yale University Press, 1955), p. 45.

231: **"You mustn't remember! . . ."**—Ibid., p. 86.

231: **"EDMUND . . ."**—Ibid., p. 174.

231: **"Something I need terribly. . . ."**—Ibid., p. 173.

232: **"The 'it' of which I speak . . ."**—Quoted in Henry James, *Notes of a Son and Brother,* in *Autobiography,* ed. F. W. Dupee (New York: Criterion, 1956), p. 510.

233: **"Such institutions as the Berghof . . ."**—Thomas Mann, "The Making of *The Magic Mountain,*" in *The Magic Mountain* (New York: Vintage, 1969), p. 719.

234: **"Can you see the hilus glands? . . ."**—Mann, *The Magic Mountain,* p. 217.

235: **"But that was no proper uniform . . ."**—Ibid., pp. 680–81.

236: **"It was . . . a fever of matter . . ."**—Ibid., pp. 275, 283–84.

237: **"As the anaesthetizing needle . . ."**—A. E. Ellis, *The Rack* (Boston: Little, Brown, 1959), pp. 139–40.

239: ***My Darling Clementine. . . .***—Directed by John Ford, screenplay by Samuel G. Engel and Winston Miller (20th Century-Fox, 1946).

241: **"Then I washed the blood . . ."**—Erich Maria Remarque, *Three Comrades,* tr. A. W. Wheen (Boston: Little, Brown, 1937), p. 480.

242: **"PAT (very low) . . ."**—F. Scott Fitzgerald, *Three Comrades,* ed. Matthew J. Bruccoli (Carbondale: Southern Illinois University Press, 1978), p. 250.

242: **"toward whatever lies ahead."**—Ibid., p. 251.

Chapter Nine: "The Haunted Hospital": Antibiotics and the Closing of the Sanatoriums

page

245: **"41 Park Ave. . . ."**—MS letter, New York State Archives, Albany, N.Y. (series 10415, box 1, folder 3M).

247: **By 1900–1904, . . .**—Statistics from Erhardt and Berlin, eds., *Mortality and Morbidity in the United States,* pp. 21–22.

247: **"We have a bare existence . . ."**—MS letter, New York State Archives, Albany, N.Y. (series 10415, box 1, folder 3M).

247: **the falloff rate doubled.**—See Mandell, Douglas, and Bennett, *Principles and Practice of Infectious Diseases,* p. 1385.

250: **"The 1880s was the decade of the bacillus, . . ."** —A[llen] K. K[rause], editorial, *American Review of Tuberculosis,* March 1917, p. 51.

250: **"We no longer look . . ."**—Ibid.

251: **"The lung . . . becomes consumptive . . ."**—Quoted in R. Y. Keers, *Pulmonary Tuberculosis: A Journey Down the Centuries* (London: Bailliere, Tindall, 1978), p. 112.

252: **"a thorough knowledge . . ."**—Ibid., p. 115.

252: **In 1937 between 50 and 80 percent . . .**—See John Alexander, *The Collapse Therapy of Pulmonary Tuberculosis* (Springfield, Illinois: C. C. Thomas, 1937), p. 3.

253: **"I felt the prick of the hypodermic needle, . . ."** —Betty MacDonald, *The Plague and I,* p. 152.

255: **Its proponents claimed . . .**—See Keers, op. cit., p. 170. Keers gives a full account of the various surgical procedures against tuberculosis that evolved in the years following World War I.

256: **A cautious and cautionary 1935 study . . .**—Andrew Peters, et al., "A Survey of Artificial Pneumothorax in Representative American Tuberculosis Sanatoria, 1915–1930," *American Review of Tuberculosis,* January 1935, pp. 85–104.

256: **"DR. JONES . . ."**—American Trudeau Society, "Present Concepts of Antimicrobial Therapy in Pulmonary Tuberculosis: Report of a Panel Discussion," etc., *American Review of Tuberculosis,* November 1953, p. 829.

256: **As early as 1941 . . .**—See Keers, op. cit., p. 162.

257: **"The pneumothorax needle . . ."**—Ibid., p. 158.

257: **"had a rigid outlook . . ."**—Ernest Chain, "A Short History of the Penicillin Discovery from Fleming's Early Observations in 1929 to the Present Time," in *The History of Antibiotics: A Symposium,* ed. John Parascandola (Madison, Wis.: American Institute of the History of Pharmacy, 1980), pp. 17–18.

258: **"The guinea pigs . . ."**—From an abstract of an article in the *New York Medical Journal,* quoted in the *American Review of Tuberculosis,* April 1918, p. 114.

259: **"Now why are these germs . . ."**—Boris D. Sokoloff, *The Story of Penicillin* (New York: Ziff-Davis, 1945), p. 4. My account of Metchnikoff's research follows Sokoloff.

260: **"When I saw the bacteria fading . . ."**—Ibid., p. 20.

261: **firmly asserted that she had seen the tubercle bacillus . . .**—McClintock, *We Take to Bed,* pp. 33–34.

263: **experiments dating back to the years . . .**—See Selman A. Waksman, *The Conquest of Tuberculosis* (Berkeley: University of California Press, 1964), p. 104.

264: **"they were deliberately set aside . . ."**—Emil Bogen, "The Treatment of Tuberculosis with Streptomycin: A Review of 110 Patients," in *Streptomycin and Dihydrostreptomycin in Tuberculosis*, eds. H. McL. Riggins and H. C. Hinshaw (New York: National Tuberculosis Association, 1949), p. 107.

264: **"quite disproportionate . . ."**—Ibid., p. 109.

264: **At the Trudeau Sanatorium, . . .**—See William Steenken, "Streptomycin and the Tubercle Bacillus," in Riggins and Hinshaw, op. cit., p. 45.

266: **"There has been no clear indication . . ."**—American Trudeau Society, "The Need for Rest Therapy in Connection with Long Courses of Drug Treatment in Pulmonary Tuberculosis: A Statement by the Committee on Therapy," *American Review of Tuberculosis,* May 1953, p. 679.

267: *"Case 3* (K.R.) . . ."—Edward H. Robitzek and Irving V. Selikoff, "Hydrazine Derivatives of Isonicotinic Acid," *American Review of Tuberculosis,* April 1952, pp. 413–18.

268: **a 1953 study concluded, . . .**—G. B. Mackaness and N. Smith, "The Bactericidal Action of Isoniazid, Streptomycin, and Terramycin on Extracellular and Intracellular Tubercle Bacilli," *American Review of Tuberculosis,* March 1953, p. 322.

268: **told by H. Herbert Fox, . . .**—See H. H. Fox, "The Chemical Approach to the Control of Tuberculosis," *Science,* 8 August 1952, pp. 129–34.

270: **"Only the recumbent figure . . ."**—*Life,* December 27, 1954, p. 76.

271: **In Kansas City, . . .**—The following material is based on an interview with Marshall Watson and Dinah Knot, November 1986.

272: **" 'You will last till to-morrow,' . . ."**—Murger, "Francine and Her Muff," *Bohemian Life,* p. 171.

Chapter Ten: Illness Imagined

page

273: **"My meeting dead corpses . . ."**—Samuel Pepys, *The Shorter Pepys,* ed. Robert Latham (Berkeley: University of California Press, 1985), pp. 526–27. I have slightly modernized the passage here.

274: **"Aged . . ."**—Facsimile in D. L. Cowen and A. B. Segelman, *Antibiotics in Historical Perspective* (Rahway, N.J.: Merck, 1981), p. 31.

276: **"Trying to comprehend . . ."**—Susan Sontag, *Illness as Metaphor* (New York: Farrar, Straus and Giroux, 1978), p. 82.

277: **"Frank Williams . . ."**—Quoted in Keers, *Pulmonary Tuberculosis: A Journey Down the Centuries,* p. 98.

280: **"I have had ample opportunity . . ."**—Trudeau, *An Autobiography,* p. 74.

282: **Such, certainly, is the tenor . . .**—See, for example, Michel Foucault, *The Birth of the Clinic: An Archaeology of Medical Perception,* tr. A. M. Sheridan Smith (New York: Vintage, 1975), pp. 196–99.

285: **"Verbally I don't learn anything . . ."**—Quoted in Sontag, op. cit., p. 7.

285: **"It was fortunate for himself . . ."**—*Journal of the Outdoor Life,* December 1908, p. 389.

286: **"Heaven forbid . . ."**—See above, p. 316 and note.

287: **"The bounds of the horizon . . ."**—P. O. Hooper, M.D., "President's Address," *Transactions of the American Medical Association* (1882), p. 97.

287: **"didn't believe much in 'germs.' "**—Trudeau, op. cit., p. 175.

Index

Index

Index

MARK CALDWELL was born in Troy, New York, in 1946. He received B.A. degrees from Fordham University and Trinity College, Cambridge, and his Ph.D. in English from Harvard University. A frequent contributor to the *Village Voice* and coeditor (with Walter Kendrick) of *The Treasury of English Poetry,* he currently teaches English at Fordham and lives in New York City.